Joanna Cholewa

Rehabilitation in Parkinson's disease

Joanna Cholewa

Rehabilitation in Parkinson's disease

LAP LAMBERT Academic Publishing

Impressum / Imprint
Bibliografische Information der Deutschen Nationalbibliothek: Die Deutsche Nationalbibliothek verzeichnet diese Publikation in der Deutschen Nationalbibliografie; detaillierte bibliografische Daten sind im Internet über http://dnb.d-nb.de abrufbar.
Alle in diesem Buch genannten Marken und Produktnamen unterliegen warenzeichen-, marken- oder patentrechtlichem Schutz bzw. sind Warenzeichen oder eingetragene Warenzeichen der jeweiligen Inhaber. Die Wiedergabe von Marken, Produktnamen, Gebrauchsnamen, Handelsnamen, Warenbezeichnungen u.s.w. in diesem Werk berechtigt auch ohne besondere Kennzeichnung nicht zu der Annahme, dass solche Namen im Sinne der Warenzeichen- und Markenschutzgesetzgebung als frei zu betrachten wären und daher von jedermann benutzt werden dürften.

Bibliographic information published by the Deutsche Nationalbibliothek: The Deutsche Nationalbibliothek lists this publication in the Deutsche Nationalbibliografie; detailed bibliographic data are available in the Internet at http://dnb.d-nb.de.
Any brand names and product names mentioned in this book are subject to trademark, brand or patent protection and are trademarks or registered trademarks of their respective holders. The use of brand names, product names, common names, trade names, product descriptions etc. even without a particular marking in this work is in no way to be construed to mean that such names may be regarded as unrestricted in respect of trademark and brand protection legislation and could thus be used by anyone.

Coverbild / Cover image: www.ingimage.com

Verlag / Publisher:
LAP LAMBERT Academic Publishing
ist ein Imprint der / is a trademark of
OmniScriptum GmbH & Co. KG
Heinrich-Böcking-Str. 6-8, 66121 Saarbrücken, Deutschland / Germany
Email: info@lap-publishing.com

Herstellung: siehe letzte Seite /
Printed at: see last page
ISBN: 978-3-659-75554-5

Copyright © 2015 OmniScriptum GmbH & Co. KG
Alle Rechte vorbehalten. / All rights reserved. Saarbrücken 2015

TABLE OF CONTENTS

Introduction	3
I. Parkinson's Disease	5
1. Epidemiology	5
2. Etiology	7
3. Symptoms	8
4. Characteristic of a sick person	10
II. Rehabilitation in Parkinson's disease	12
1. Pharmacological treatment, surgical treatment, and rehabilitation	12
2. Quality of life	13
3. Basics of rehabilitation	14
4. Rehabilitation treatment of main symptoms	16
5. Planning of motor rehabilitation	19
6. The research problem in literature	24
III. The aim of the study and research questions	26
IV. Material and research methods	27
1. Characteristic of the subjects	27
2. Methods and tools of the research	28
3. Research procedure	30
4. Methods of research material analyses	31
V. The results	31
1. Descriptive statistics of ability level in performing daily actives prior to the experiment	32
2. Effect of rehabilitation on efficiency in performing daily activities	36
3. Response of PD patients to exercises depending on the selected factors	47
4. Discussion	49
5. Conclusions	56
Reference	57
Appendix	68

Introduction

Parkinson's disease (PD) is one of the most common diseases of the central nervous system. It does not shorten the life expectancy but makes living more difficult. We meet people suffering from this disease in a mild form almost every day in the street, not realizing that the person with stooped posture, slower movements, trembling hands struggles with Parkinson's disease. People with advanced Parkinson's disease are rarely seen, disorder eliminates them from everyday life. Difficulties with walking are so great that consequently lead to leaving home less and less often. They stop contacting with friends, and feel embarrassed by their behaviour and appearance.

Due to demographic trends to gradual aging of the population, the number of people affected by Parkinson's disease is gradually increasing, requiring continual and longstanding pharmacological and non-pharmacological therapy. Progression of the disease requires greater and greater involvement of close family in the care of a sick person. It is important that all the patient, family and carer have as much factual information as possible about Parkinson's disease, its causes, symptoms, treatment options and the need for constant physical activity.

Despite much greater opportunities of symptomatic treatment, the progression of the disease cannot be stopped. A complete understanding of the disease with its entire symptomatology of movement disorders, careful observation and analysis, collaboration with patient, cooperation with groups of specialists from various fields can help maintain the quality of life at a better level. Rehabilitation is one of the factors that can help patients maintain higher efficiency and allow them to function better every day.

The paper presents rehabilitation treatment options. It is worth noting that intensive and extensive research on the causes and more effective methods of treatment are being carried out worldwide. Research conducted in this study aimed at providing improvement in the quality of life of patients with PD by the selection of appropriate exercises. Despite the progression of the disease and associated limitations, patients engaged in rehabilitation activities can enjoy the fullness of personal and professional life for many years.

People with Parkinson's disease are not left to their fate. Both they and their carers can ask the Association of People with Parkinson's Disease for help and advice. A number of people interested in cooperation and in need of support is increasing. Association support patients and their families, provide educational materials, conduct lectures about important issues related to the disease, organize rehabilitation activities and self-help groups for patients and people involved in taking care of them.

I. Parkinson's Disease

1. Epidemiology

Parkinson's disease (PD) is after Alzheimer's disease the second most frequent degenerative disease of the nervous system. It occurs worldwide and affects all populations. It is estimated that it affects about 0.3% of the general population, increasing with age to 1.4% in people over 55 years of age and to 3.4% after 75 years. Its prevalence is estimated at 120-180 people per 100,000 in temperate climates. The first symptoms show up most often between 50 and 60 years old. The disease can also begin before the age of 40, and affects approximately 5-10% of patients and is a challenge for clinicians.

The first information about the PD comes from the turn of the fifteenth and sixteenth centuries. Defined by Leonardo Da Vinci. In his notes he wrote about "people whose soul cannot control the movements even if they take an extreme form of continual tremor "[Paty 2001]. In 1817, James Parkinson (1755-1827), published a paper: *An Essay on the Shaking Palsy* describing strange disease, calling it paralysis agitans. This paper was the beginning of all subsequent research on the disease. Jean Martin Charkot did not agree with the term used by Parkinson's – "paralysis agitans", and he first proposed naming the disease after James Parkinson, noting that in this disease there is no paralysis and tremor may not always appear. To prevail over the midbrain by the disease process was described in 1895 by a Charkot's student - Brossaud, and confirmed later in the 20s by Tretiakoff. In 1912, Lewy described the cellular inclusions, named after Lewy body. Joseph Babinski first described oscillations in clinical status of patients, now known as fluctuations. Parkinson's disease is the most common form of so-called parkinsonism, that is a group of diseases with a similar clinical picture and similar symptoms. Its exact cause is not [Diamond et al. 1990, Friedman, Barcikowska 1994, Playfer 1999].

Taking into consideration the aging of the population, it can be expected that by 2020 over 40 million people worldwide will have been suffering from a chronic neurological disease, becoming then more and more serious medical and social problem for patients, their families and carers. The very process of aging of the human body carries a number of disorders and impairments of psychomotor performance, and combined with PD, especially in the later stages, is associated with a number of restrictions in patient's life, causing gradual loss of independence and a reduced quality of life. Then a restriction of independence in performing simple life activities such as dressing, eating, personal hygiene follows. This occurs in 50% of patients with PD, compared to 13.2% in the group of healthy individuals. In the performance of complex tasks such as the use of phone, shopping, transportation, medication, restriction occurs in 80% of patients with PD compared to 28% of the testing population. Much more often we placed patients in nursing homes (about 20%) and about 4.5% of healthy ones. The degree of dependence of patients on the environment is a cause of immediate family involvement in the care of the patient. Requirements and commitment increase with the progression of the disease and are associated with symptoms of both mobility and immobility. Attitude of the family and the environment is also affecting course of the disease. Appropriate information and awareness of the nature of the disease, its basics, and also many additional symptoms, allow to effectively eliminate obstacles and threats.

2. Etiology

Neuropathological base of PD is a progressive loss of dopamine-generating cells in the substantia nigra, damage to dopamine-generating pathway and secondary changes in dopamine receptors. Neuropathological exponent of PD are Lewy bodies consisting mainly of abnormally folded accumulation of the α-synuclein protein. Degenerative process leads to a decrease in dopamine levels in the nigrostriatial pathway and clinical manifestation of the disease. Motor symptoms appear at the level of deficiency approximately 60% to 70%.

The etiology of PD remains unknown. Genetic predispositions are taken into account, that are leading to beginning of the programmed apoptosis or premature aging, phenomenon of oxidative stress, contribution of neurotoxin endogenous or exogenous neurotoxic substances, deficiency of growth factors, glutamate-induced excitotoxicity, disorders of endogenous neuroprotective processes, inflammatory agents.

With respect to the etiology of Parkinson's disease, there is evidence for participation of both environmental and genetic factors, but so far a specific cause of the disease has not been detected.

PD, despite the significant progress in the treatment, increases mortality in a population of patients. The standardized mortality rate for patients with Parkinson's disease in Norway is 1.5 regardless of gender and age of onset.

For many years, people have been trying to determine if there are risk factors for PD. According to most assessments, the only known risk factor is age, because together with age the present of Lewy bodies increases.

Despite of the intensive researches the reasons of the disease and its pathogenesis are not clearly defined so far. Also the searches on how to prevent or inhibit the pace of development of PD have not given measurable results.

3. Symptoms

The first symptoms are nonspecific: weakness, tiredness, easy fatigability, because of that PD can be undiagnosed for a long time. Only when we have more specific symptoms the neurologist can diagnose properly.

The most common symptoms occurring in PD are:
- tremor of hands, arms, legs, jaw and face,
- rigidity of limbs and torso,
- bradykinesia,
- impaired postural reflexes.

Consequently, together with the development of the disease the symptoms are becoming more severe, there are difficulty with walking, speaking and performance of simple life tasks. Tremor of hands remaining at rest is observed in 75% of patients and initially occurs most frequently in one hand. Asymmetry of symptoms is a characteristic of PD. The first symptom of PD may also be the malfunction of one hand, manifested by difficulty in fasten buttons or writing. Sometimes the disease begins with a dystonic posture of one upper limb.

Another fairly rare first symptom occurring more frequently in young patients are pains - like root pains of one limb, which later appear with parkinsonian tremor and rigidity.

One of the first symptoms may also be changes in speaking, characterized by a reduction of the amplitude of the movement of facial muscles, therefore hipomimia and limiting the amplitude of the vocal cords movement, leading to characteristic patient speech - monotonous, "flattened" and without intonation. Typical of other expressions of the amplitude limitations of movement is also micrograph (changes in writing, that become small and tiny) and difficulty in tipping from side to side in bed, walking trouble, as well as the initiation of the first step. In addition to motor symptoms, the onset of the disease may be present as a vegetative symptoms such as constipation, drooling, seborrhea. These symptoms are often accompanied by depression.

The most troublesome are so-called primary symptoms of PD: muscle rigidity, tremor, bradykinesia and poverty of movements, difficulty with balance and walking.

In some patients secondary symptoms appear. Some of them result from the influence of one or more primary symptoms for a given muscle group. For example, difficulties in speech are the result of rigidity, tremor and poverty throat muscle movements. Sometimes secondary symptoms may be more onerous than the primary. Apart from the difficulty in speaking, these include: depression, difficulty with falling asleep and easy waking up, dementia, drooling and difficulty with swallowing, constipation and weight loss. Less frequently occurring symptoms are symptoms such as dystonic, for example blepharospasm, expressing the inability to open the closed eyes lids or keep them open, which makes it more difficult to perform many daily activities.

The diagnosis of PD is a clinical diagnosis, based on the finding of resting tremor, bradykinesia and/or akinesia (inability of the movements), muscle rigidity, the presence of symptoms such as postural instability, characteristic unilateral onset of symptoms and the exclusion of symptomatic parkinsonism and finding a good clinical response to drugs that stimulate the dopaminergic system. Helpful in establishing the diagnosis may be additional symptoms such as vegetative disorders: drooling, seborrhea, sweating attacks, respiratory disorders, sleep disturbances, orthostatic hypotension, constipation, potency disorders, the symptoms of bulbar: dysarthria and dysphagia, cognitive disorders: dementia, depression and pain.

The diagnosis of PD, especially in its early stages, can be a difficult task, even though the disease is so-called the diseases "recognizable on the street." Outside motor symptoms, although that they are not dominating in the clinical picture of Parkinson's disease, they can significantly affect the quality of life for both the patients themselves and their carers. Helpful in the diagnosis of PD are generally accepted by UK Parkinson's Disease Society Brain Bank clinical criteria that allow for the correct diagnosis.

4. Characteristic of a sick person

A typical profile of a person with PD, referred to so-called "stooped posture", is widely described in the scientific literature. Depending on the duration and severity of the disease in varying degrees, expressed changes are characterized by:
- forward ejecting the neck and head,
- forward bending of the thoracic spine,
- flattening of the physiological lordosis of the lumbar spine,
- setting shoulder joints in extensor position, adduction and rotation to the inside,
- setting elbows in the flexion position with pronation,
- setting radial-carpal joints in neutral position or palmar flexion and ulnar abduction,
- slight bend fingers in the metacarpophalangeal joints and interphalangeal straightening,
- setting the thumb in a position of adduction,
- slight flexion, abduction and internal rotation of hip joints,
- a slight bend in the knee joints,
- tendency to dorsiflexion of the upper part of ankle.

As the disease progresses we can add the postural instability, impaired autonomic nervous system and a variety of symptoms of disorders of nervous system and mental disorders (depression, agitation, confusion, cognitive impairment and dementia). Subjective complaints include difficulty in movement, tremor, muscle cramps, imbalance, often severe persistent pain, depression and sleep disorders. If left untreated Parkinson's disease causes a 2-5 times increase in mortality, clearly associated with the severity of the disease.

Quality of life deteriorates significantly with increasing degree of disability, severity of depression level, and dementia and treatment costs. According to the regression analysis, the variables with the greatest predictive value for the quality of life were: depression and the occurrence of motor fluctuations.

Falls are the leading cause of mortality, disability and the need to place patients in a nursing home. The causes of falls are diverse: abnormal posture and gait, muscle rigidity, symptomatic orthostatic hypotension, motor fluctuations (dyskinesia), syndrome of sudden deterioration ("on-off", with episodes of sudden "solidify" or "freezing") and finally dementia. They concern particularly patients with advanced disease. In proceedings healing involves primarily the optimization of treatment, physical rehabilitation and education of patients and their families.

II. Rehabilitation in Parkinson's disease

1. Pharmacological treatment, surgery treatment, and rehabilitation

The disease is treated symptomatically with progression in pharmacology, medicaments are better tolerated by the body of the patient, more effectively reduce the symptoms of the disease, and at the same time producing fewer side effects.

The development of neurosurgery, has created a new method of treatment by surgery, they are used effectively eliminating or greatly reducing mainly tremor.

Regardless of the method, the rehabilitation is an integral part of the treatment process, and through its own characteristics (complexity, different stages, regularity), embraces the whole person in a changing treatment methods and recovery. Rehabilitation is not only a way to restore lost of psychophysical performance during disease, but it is also a form of secondary prevention. It is a process involving all areas of rehabilitation (including speech and swallowing disorders, psychological problems, the ability to work, social and living things, etc.). In these proceedings stand permanent priorities: self-service, self-reliance, locomotion. Doing so may significantly determine the quality of life of patients.

2. Quality of life

The World Health Organization already in 1949, defined quality of life as a state of complete physical, mental and social wellbeing and not merely the absence of disease. Currently a WHO definition of quality of life as the perception of unit and her life position in the context of the culture and value system surrounding unit in relation to its goals, expectations and standards [WHO 1992] is promoted.

This issue is particularly important for patients with PD, because the solid accumulation of disease symptoms substantially affect the quality of life. The main therapeutic actions are aimed at the most favorable reduction of symptoms.

3. Basics of rehabilitation

Symptomatology of idiopathic PD is the expression of complex disorders of brain structures in activities that play an important role not only in the planning, initiation of movement, but also in the integration of external stimuli and control activities attention. It is worthy to emphasize that it is not only one dimension disorder - "mechanical", but the fact of taking the disease process of the whole person of the patient in a broader sense all of their activities. Hence, we can pull out of the above symptoms several conclusions which should be considered during rehabilitation treatment if treatment is to be effective.

Initiative and motivation - about 40% of patients have depression, because of that willingness to cooperate can be significantly reduced. Psychiatric disorders are often severe by impaired mobility, that is, moving difficulty. Assigning outside contact and well structured in terms of visual surroundings simplify the cooperation of the patient much more than a well-thought-out warning and advice appealing to the patient's own initiative.

Learning the moves - in the early stage of the disease, there is a weakening of the ability to learn, while memory of the events and memory of the verbal material (declarative memory) is not impaired. This means that in practice the patient is not able to learn new movement patterns, or he/she is doing it with great difficulty. Also, do not expect that the new exercises which the patient learnt during the rehabilitation will be repeated at home by himself/herself. In further stages of the disease, when we have to add declarative memory impairment, the patient does not remember the verbal instructions for physical exercises.

Stability during standing and walking - because of impaired balance symptom there is a significant degree of impairment of walking and standing. Because patients are not able to predict or control the falling down, they become fearful and uncertain, which further increase senility. Therefore, patient should start with regular and intense balance exercise. The goal is to train the trigger skill that is an adequate balance response to the destabilization of the position, as well as the ability of noticing and correcting deviations of posture.

Comprehensive motor programs - in an advanced stage of the disease there is an inability to perform two simultaneous motor actions. Complex motor system should be decomposed into its constituent parts, which will be performed one after the other. In everyday life, these conditions are clearly present in the situation, for example, when patient is removing the keys from a coat pocket, while he/she is moving. Thus, during rehabilitation process patient should practice situations that require a comprehensive, simultaneous motor actions (also with only one hand), and what is more important in the early stages of the disease.

Programs of automated or repetitive movements - rhythmic - in PD it becomes impossible to perform repeated rhythmic motor scheme. This can be seen especially in the case of gait disorder in advanced stage where the absence of an external rhythm transmission, the frequency and length of steps decreases. The problem is the difficulty in obtaining internal rhythm or disorder of taking this rhythm into account in planning of locomotor activity. It is therefore advisable, in the process of rehabilitation to exercise external rhythm broadcasting.

Internal control of motor programs - pathology in PD relates to anatomic structures in the nervous system that are responsible for the conduct and control of free movements internally generated. Hence, it is important to prepare the visual environment so that the patient may be able to moving around better and somehow "hold firmly". As the system of deliberated moves is impoverishing pretty fast (hypokinesia), the compensation strategy is possible; the patient is recommended to plan deliberate movements, conscious kind of over scaling.

Because movement disorders are a special feature of PD and may significantly affect individual ability to perform learned motor actions, such as walking, writing, rotation, and putting to bed and getting up from bed, because of that the main task of the physiotherapist is to teach people with PD strategies of coping with handicaps and disability. These strategies should allow for easier movement, minimize disability and maintain independence in everyday life.

4. Rehabilitation treatment of the main symptoms

Physical exercises are very important as a supportive treatment for the treatment of PD, often becoming one of the most beneficial forms of activity for the patient. A very important factor that increases the chances of success in the rehabilitation of people with PD is the awareness of risks posed by the disease. This awareness is all the more necessary as the disease develops slowly and can be easy to overlook the negative changes that increase year by year. A person with PD gradually gets used to the progressive restriction, not realizing that she/he can counteract them. Common symptoms in PD are resting tremor, and increased muscle tension, which, because of its origin is called extrapyramidal rigidity. Methods that are used are the following: autogenic training, progressive muscle stretching according to Jacobs, as well as some breathing exercises. Resting tremor largely disappears during sleep and is dependent on the emotional state of the individual patient, which probably explains the beneficial effects of relaxing exercises.

Ad hoc the best results in the treatment of rigidity are achieved through the use of heat treatments, particularly treatments in the aquatic environment: hydro massage, whirlpool massage, exercises performed in warm water. A typical symptom of PD is also so called impoverishment of the movement, which is expressed as a decrease in range of motion performed independently by the patient that are referring to active movements. A manifestation of the impoverishment of the movement is also bradykinesia, or slow the pace of the movement and the delayed response of the originating action in response to a stimulus. Another symptom is to reduce the amplitude of active movement during repetitive tasks. This symptom is decisive, for example, for a walk, which is a typical example of repetitive tasks.

These symptoms pose a threat to the formation of contractures and perpetuating negative consequences for flexible movement system elements, or muscles, and ligaments and joint capsules. Risk awareness of the formation of contractures should be accompanied by all patients from the time of diagnosis of PD, finding out about their disease. Admission to the formation of contractures brings with it a number of far-reaching consequences. Contracture of the shoulder girdle muscle and shoulder muscles lead to rounding up the back, which adversely affects the function of the spine, hence the common pain syndromes of the cervical spine and borderline cervical - thoracic. Is also reduced mobility of the chest, which affects badly lungs ventilation, resulting in deteriorating respiratory function and overall condition. Muscle contractures of the lower limbs - hip flexor, knee and ankle lead to difficulties already disturbed gait. Make that step becomes even shorter, more trailing, on a narrower basis. The muscles of the hands and forearms deserve special attention, which contracture can significantly limit the dexterity of hands. In the prophylaxis of contractures, stretching exercises and stretching positions at risk muscle groups are playing a leading role. Based on the assessment of ranges of the movement of both active and passive joints, physiotherapists can specify individual mobility limitations and prepare a set of stretching exercises.

Another symptom consisting of the impoverishment of the movement is counter-rotation disorder. It consists of opposing the abolition of the proper motion of the shoulder girdle in relation to the movement of pelvic girdle. In normal conditions this mechanism is observed during gait and manifests itself in the forward swing arm opposite to the front leg. It also helps for example in situations such as turning in bed, when to change the position we are supporting on the shoulders and turning the hips, or (more often) the opposite: first we turn the shoulders and hips are the fulcrum for the movement. Disturbance of this reflex is the cause of apraxia axis, the impossibility of turning around the long axis of the body. This, in turn, makes it difficult for operations such as changing the direction of walking, turning around in a standing position, or self-change position in bed. Counteraction of this problem, is the inclusion of a set of general development exercises, movements of the elements of a comprehensive turns individual body segments: head, shoulders of the rim shoulder, torso, hips and lower limbs. The movements should be sweeping and freely, which promotes muscle relaxation. An important element of these exercises is clear "check" the fulcrum, for example when turning the hips to the left in the supine position firmly, and even overly tight, push the right elbow by pushing it into the ground.

Very wide issue related to PD is the problem of smooth, and efficient gait. Gait disturbances in advanced forms of the disease are so frequent and so typical that operates the term "parkinsonian gait." It is characterized by the following elements: a slow pace, reduced mobility in all joints of the lower limbs manifested by shortening step, feet wandering and narrow base, the abolition of co-movements manifested by a lack of arm swings, difficult to start walking and stopping it, frequent loss of balance and falls, so-called tunnel symptom and freezing stage. These disorders are a very serious problem in life and rehabilitation.

5. Planning of motor rehabilitation

In the first 10 years of the disease, patients frequently exhibit bradykinesia, mild hypokinesia during walking, resting tremor, micrograph and mute of speech. It is believed that in later stages the following ones become bigger problems: accelerating steps, dyskinesia, severe hypokinesia, akinesia (freezing), postural instability and falls. One of the features of PD, is that there is no loss of the movement, but rather the problems with its activation.

The neurological rehabilitation is using the algorithm for effective rehabilitation more than other sectors of rehabilitations. Diagnostics - estimation of prognosis - functional estimation - rehabilitation planning - realization. It means a fixed sequence of stages of the rehabilitation.

The needs and the range patients rehabilitation with Parkinson's disease is determined for each patient individually, using the Unified Parkinson Disease Rating Scale (UPDRS). The basis for improvement are: physiotherapy, for example therapeutic exercises and teaching activities of daily living. Also important are: occupational therapy, speech therapy, hydrotherapy, thermotherapy, relaxation training, choreotherapy, music therapy, art therapy, walking, hiking, games and physical fun, recreation (swimming, table tennis, cycling, billiards, bowling, karate and yoga elements), psychotherapy.

The role of the physiotherapist is to plan an exercise program that is adapted to the changing capabilities of patients and their caregivers. The current model developed for the purpose of physiotherapy of people with PD is based on the assumption that the proper motions can be achieved by teaching patients an avoidance strategy "the pathology of the basal ganglia." During the planning of rehabilitation, therapists should take into account:

- reaction of movement disorders on external conditions and strategies related to the concentration
- knowledge of that how treatments can be adapted, adapting them to the severity of cognitive impairment,

- the need for performance analysis in the performance of functional tasks as a basis for planning the task of training programs,
- drug effects on movement disorders.

In the rehabilitation of people with PD are valid universal canons of rehabilitation. Complexity (anastomosis) indicates that rehabilitation team is performing these tasks. Planning for rehabilitation must be preceded by a thorough diagnosis and evaluation of prognosis. Aspects such as neurological condition, severity of the disease and the patient's mental state should be taken into account. Do not forget that the process of treatment, including rehabilitation, is primarily aimed at improving the quality of life of the patient. Planning for rehabilitation should be focused on the needs and capabilities of the patient, taking into account his/her preferences and expectations. It should also take into account the risks, particularly the risk of fall. Planning must be done with the active participation of the patient and patient's family, and should therefore take into account the family's participation in the whole process of rehabilitation and its goals should be agreed upon and accepted by both the patient and his/her family.

A very important task for physiotherapists is, that in the case of starting PD, through regular exercise they should strive to overcome the basic symptoms: hypokinesia, rigidity and tremor, so patient will be able to maintain a normal life and professional activities as long as possible. At later stage, rehabilitation should delay the state of dependence by supporting the independence movement.

During planning the physiotherapy programs customized to the individual needs of the patient and their caregivers, physiotherapists should consider the impact of aging, co morbidities and secondary adaptive changes in skeletal-muscular system and cardiovascular system. Despite considerable difficulties caused by disorders such as hypokinesia, akinesia and dyskinesia, people with PD in certain circumstances, have the ability to move quickly from almost normal dimension of the movement. When patient perform simple tasks such as pointing ballistic object or catching a flying ball - the range and speed of the movement are often correct. However, when combining simple movements in a long and complex sequences of operations, the patient performs them slowly and with much greater difficulty. Ability to perform the movements can be improved by teaching people with PD, divide long or complicated sequences into component parts and focus on the performance of each part separately. Patients with PD benefit by focusing on doing one task at a time and avoid performing dual tasks. Preparation of the scheduled movement in advance by using thoughts and visualization of this movement may also be beneficial for patient. There are collected evidence that people with PD can move more easily when someone provided them outside signals that can "control" performance of the movements. Signals can be either visual or auditory. Auditory signals are most effective in patients with akinesia of gait, and phenomenon of "freezing", and visual signals are most effective in patients with hypokinesia of gait. The rhythmic sensory signals may be useful as an aid in starting activities such as walking. Exercises in the final stage of PD may be less effective because patients show a reduced ability to learn new motor exercises.

In physiotherapy, exercises can be carried out individually or in groups, and should be adjusted to the severity of the disease. Also there is conduct of breathing exercises, stretching, general development, practicing of getting up from a sitting position, learning how to walk, hands exercise, facial muscles exercises, rhythmic exercises connected with music, exercise with special equipment (stick, ball, etc.). Coordination and balance exercises by H. S. Frenkel.

Any kind of daily activity gives gladness, satisfaction and meaning of life, but to implement it as long as it is possible the regular exercises have to be performed. Even regular movement, but with the same character, does not protect a man with PD against the negative effects of the disease. A set of exercises to improve should be designed so as to take into account all essential aspects of the proper functioning of the musculoskeletal system. If the correct functioning is no longer possible because of the fixed "cavities", then exercise should take into account the current state of the patient's motor abilities. Therefore, it is necessary to have regular contact with a therapist who can assess a functional status of the patient and according to this estimation, she/he can develop an appropriate set of exercises.

Proceedings to improve must take into account all the human motor skills: flexibility, strength, speed, endurance, agility and motor coordination. It is also necessary to adjust the manner of improvement, taking into account elements such as age, duration of disease, the overall physical condition as an expression of endurance cardio - respiratory, other chronic comorbidities (coronary heart disease, hypertension, osteoarthritis of the limbs and spine, and other), severity of illness, acquired and fixed secondary complications and their stage (for example, contractures of joints and muscles, breathing disorders) and the current progress of rehabilitation.

For efficient use of the rehabilitation effort that accompanies by rehabilitation it is necessary to follow some basic rules:

1. The physical condition of the patient may fluctuate during the day, not least because of medication. For exercise therapist should choose a time of day when the mood is better,
2. Patients with PD often have depression, therefore the self-making effort exceed their mental capabilities. In this kind of situations the initiative and motivation rests with the physiotherapist,
3. The PD is a neurodegenerative disease and thus some of the functions and capabilities of the nervous system tend to be lost permanently. Therefore, rehabilitation should strive not to restore lost function, but to improve and maintain those functions that are still existing,
4. In the early stages of the disease it should be encouraged to engage in complex activities and in advanced disease - vice versa - teach break down complex tasks for simpler elements, for example: as long as possible, getting out of bed the patient should perform in one smooth motion from a lying to sitting and the standing, but during the advanced PD divided into "segments movement",
5. In the early stages of the disease we should focus on combining activities (for example: transfer of the object from hand to hand,

conversation, etc.). While in advanced PD, concentrate on proper rhythmic gait,
6. Use an external stimulation with the use of auditory, visual and tactile. For example: walking efficiency can be improved by walking to the beat of the music; walking is easier to initiate crossing located cane, or drawn line, etc.

Knowledge about the rehabilitation of people with PD is growing, but still the awareness of the need for patients rehabilitation, both among physicians, physical therapists and the patients themselves require verification. Not only physiotherapists, but also people with PD have to want to find in himself/herself desire and motivation to exercise to improve daily activities.

6. The research problem in literature

The literature on the effectiveness of physiotherapy in patients with PD there are no studies that are comparing effects of exercise based on the functional tasks of the movements. We observe a clear division of study into two groups: focusing on general issues and dealing with specific issues. In the papers, which were analyzed the improving of mobility, posture and balance, to measure of the effectiveness of physiotherapy as primary determinants, were used: walk on time, or measurements of step length. Most of the work showed an improvement of at least one of the test elements immediately after treatment. No effect was observed in the five researches that deal with patients after treatment.

The positive effect of physical exercise on some parameters in patients with PD referred to improve the efficiency of circulatory following aerobic exercise, greater achievements of fitness as a result of assisted by sensory techniques of reps compared to conventional therapy.

Available in the literature study of the effect of physiotherapy and/or occupational therapy on the functioning of patients with PD showed at least one positive change among the examined parameters. Improvement of mobility and independence was confirmed, but according to previous studies, the improvement was small or moderate. However, some authors express the view that rehabilitation proceedings do not affect the quality of patients life. No evidence of the effectiveness of rehabilitation in PD has already been noted by other researchers [Gibberd et al. 1981]. This is probably due to the differences and methodological weaknesses of the experiments, such as patient selection criteria, the lack of a control group, the use of unreliable research tools or lack of objectivity.

Although the available studies do not undermine the need for additional forms of assistance of non-pharmacological therapy such as rehabilitation, it is necessary to formulate a thesis about the importance of the rehabilitation proceedings in PD. To be able to carry out rehabilitation in this group of patients as a specific form of therapy, we have to determine the effectiveness of physiotherapy in situations where the cause of symptoms is irreversible, and for the disease process which has its base in a constantly progressive neurodegenerative changes there is no causal treatment.

Given the lack of a clear position in previous studies it was decided to carry out a study to assess the assumed efficiency improvements and at the same time to verify the view, that is not so rare, that physical therapy is not helpful in the treatment of Parkinson's disease, and if it is helpful it is a non-specific interaction [Borrione et al. 2014, Gage, Storey 2004, Goodwin et al., 2008, Tomlison et al. 2012].

III. The aim of the study and research questions

The aim of the study was to determine the effect of rehabilitation on the severity of the motor symptoms of Parkinson's disease, depending on the severity of the disease.

In the paper we assumed the specific objectives in the form of the following research questions:
1. Does regularly conducted rehabilitation cause an improvement in the motor symptoms of PD?
2. Is the response of patients with PD to exercise different depending on age, gender, disease duration and regularity of exercise?
3. Has there been an improvement in the daily activities, the degree of self-reliance?
4. Has there been an improvement in the quality of life?

The study made it possible to verify the research hypothesis:

Systematically conducted rehabilitation reduces the consequences of Parkinson's disease, allows for improvement in daily activities. Through the use of rehabilitation, the quality of life of patients with Parkinson's disease is improving.

IV. Material and research methods

1. Characteristic of the subjects

The studies involved people who gave their written consent to participate in the study after obtaining full information about the purpose and nature of research:
- with a diagnosis of PD made by a doctor specializing in the diagnosis and treatment of PD. The diagnosis was placed in accordance with the criteria of the United Kingdom Parkinson's Disease Society Brain Bank,
- in stage III of disease according to the scale of Hoehn and Yahr'a [Hoehn, Yahr 1967],
- no contraindications to performing exercise.

The exclusion criteria of the study.

Persons who were not qualified for testing:
- chronically ill patients with contraindications to performing exercise,
- no consent to participate in the study.

The subjects were divided into two groups: experimental and control. The characteristics of the subjects are presented in tab.4.1.1.

Tab.4.1.1. Characteristic of the subjects.

Group	Experimental	Control
Population	40	30
Gender Women/men	13/27	11/19
Age (years) Women/ men	71,23±5,89/ 69,70±5,73	70,36±7,15/ 70,11±4,20
Duration of disease (years) Women/ men	6,62±2,26/ 8,70±3,69	6,09±2,02/ 8,05±2,01

2. Methods and tools of the research

The study used an experimental method aimed at tracking connections and relationships of cause and effect. We used the technique of deliberate selection.

For the assessment of the severity of PD was used common scale of Hoehn and Yahr'a [1967], allowing for the estimated breakdown of the stages of PD, and relying primarily on the assessment of movement disorders. The 5-point scale ratings are characterized by different degrees:

Stage I: unilateral symptoms, no or slight weakening of activities

Stage II: bilateral symptoms, lack of imbalances,

Stage III: first symptoms of postural reflexes disorders,

Stage IV: severe symptoms,

Stadium V: needs help, uses a wheelchair.

To determine the clinical status of the patient the Unified Parkinson's Disease Rating Scale (UPDRS) Part I, II, III. [Brusse et al., 2005] was used. It is a comprehensive, global numerical scale used to assess the number of motor and behavioral symptoms of PD. Includes an estimation of mental status, estimation of ability to perform daily activities, the research of physical activities, to estimation of the potential complications of therapy. The result is the sum of the points of the corresponding parts of the scale.

Part I. Intellectual status, behavior, mood (0 - 4); memory and orientation, abnormal thinking (after taking drugs), depression, motivation/initiative.

Part II. Activities of daily living and parkinsonian signs (0 - 4, on / off): speech, salivation, swallowing, handwriting, use of cutlery, dressing up, hygiene, functioning in bed, falling, tripping (freezing), walking, tremor, sensory problems associated with PD.

Part III. Examination of the motor state (0 - 4, on/off): speech, facial expression, rest tremor, positional tremor and other type of action tremor, rigidity, alternating movements, getting up from a chair, posture, gait, stability of balance, bradykinesia general.

In addition, an estimation of daily activities we used scale of Schwab and England Activities of Daily Living (ADL). It is a numerical scale that estimates the impact of Parkinson's disease on mobility during daily activities such as: speech, swallowing, handwriting, use of cutlery during meals, dressing up, daily hygiene, turning in bed at bedtime, gait, and the occurrence and severity of some symptoms: falls, drooling, suddenly stopping while walking, tremors, movement disorders.

Also we evaluated the level of quality of life by using the PDQ-39 scale (The quality of life in Parkinson's disease). This is a subjective scale, which has a proven sensitivity, specificity and repeatability [Holbrook, Skilbeck 1983, Karlsen et al., 1999]. It consists of 39 parts by assessing quality of life and health status of patients with Parkinson's disease. The result is expressed in numerical value.

3. Research procedure

The study involved two groups of patients with Parkinson's disease: experimental group (tested) and a control group. The experimental group of patients participated in rehabilitation activities in the gym twice a week (60 min). Classes at the gym aimed at increasing the range of motion, improve balance, and improve motor skills and walking. The main emphasis was placed on the ability to cope with daily activities. In addition, subjects were given a set of exercises to be performed daily at home. Proposed sets of exercises were developed by the author of this paper based on the literature. The control group consisted of patients in the same stage of the disease, respectively, matched for age and gender, but not participating in rehabilitation activities.

In order to determine the effect of exercise on the mobility of patients in both groups a clinical assessment of research before and after their completion was performed. The study period covered 12 weeks.

4. Methods of research material analyses

In the paper the dependent variable was the efficiency of the process of rehabilitation. Independent variables were: period of illness, age, gender of respondents, the total duration of rehabilitation activities.

The obtained results were subjected to statistical analysis. There were calculated basic descriptive statistics: the arithmetic mean, standard deviation, skewness index, kurtosis. The distribution of the study groups was tested by using the Kolmogorov-Smirnov test.

To assess the significance of differences between the two groups before the experiment we used t - student test for independent samples. To assess the significance of differences between results obtained by the patients in the used scales, before and after the 12 weeks period of rehabilitation, ANOVA analysis was applied. Depending on the significance of main effects and interactions there was performed a post-hoc analysis.

5. Test results

The results were collected and statistically analyzed and presented in tables and graphs.

1. Descriptive statistics of ability level in performing daily activities prior to the experiment

Tables 5.1.1 and 5.1.2 present the statistical characteristics of the results obtained in the various tests before the experiment in the study and control groups of women.

Tab.5.1.1. Statistical characteristics of the results obtained in the various tests in the experimental group of women (EW) prior to the experiment.

Variable	$\bar{x}$	S	As	Ku
Age [y]	71,23	5,89	0,54	0,31
Period of illness	6,62	2,26	0,77	1,84
UPDRS part I [score]	3,00	1,68	1,12	1,40
UPDRS part II [score]	15,38	7,76	-0,20	-0,78
UPDRS part III [score]	22,00	9,35	-0,50	-0,72
UPDRS (I, II, III) [score]	40,38	16,99	-0,50	-1,02
Schwab & England [%]	72,31	5,99	-0,07	0,05
PDQ-39 [score]	39,00	20,44	0,34	0,70

$\bar{x}$ - mean,
S – standard deviation,
As – skweness index,
Ku – kurtosis.

Tab.5.1.2. Statistical characteristics of the results obtained in the various tests in the control group of women (CW) prior to the experiment.

Variable	$\bar{x}$	S	As	Ku
Age [y]	70,36	7,15	-1,30	3,07
Period of illness [y]	6,09	2,02	0,47	-0,05
UPDRS part I [score]	2,91	1,58	-0,75	-0,53
UPDRS part II [score]	15,91	4,44	1,10	1,57
UPDRS part III [score]	22,00	5,10	-0,48	-0,26
UPDRS (I, II, III) [score]	40,82	9,16	0,52	0,81
Schwab & England [%]	73,64	5,05	0,66	-1,96
PDQ-39 [score]	41,45	14,16	0,54	1,02

Tables 5.1.3. and 5.1.4. present the statistical characteristics of the results obtained in the various tests before the experiment in study and control groups of men.

Tab.5.1.3. Statistical characteristics of the results obtained in the various tests in the experimental group of men (EM) prior to the experiment.

Variable	$\bar{x}$	S	A_s	K_u
Age [y]	69,70	5,73	-0,07	-1,06
Period of illnesss [y]	8,70	3,69	0,81	0,13
UPDRS part I [score]	2,41	1,15	0,41	-0,65
UPDRS part II [score]	15,48	6,01	0,00	-0,48
UPDRS part III [score]	21,44	7,00	-0,15	-0,33
UPDRS (I, II, III) [score]	39,33	12,96	-0,30	-0,50
Schwab & England [%]	72,22	7,51	0,19	-0,05
PDQ-39 [score]	40,52	11,47	-0,49	-0,62

Tab.5.1.4. Statistical characteristics of the results obtained in the various tests in the control group of men (CM) prior to the experiment.

Variable	$\bar{x}$	S	A_s	K_u
Age [y]	70,11	4,20	-0,79	1,43
Period of illness [y]	8,05	2,01	0,29	-0,55
UPDRS part I [score]	2,26	1,05	0,39	-0,90
UPDRS part II [score]	15,95	5,45	0,50	-0,22
UPDRS part III [score]	21,95	6,49	0,41	-0,79
UPDRS (I, II, III) [score]	40,16	10,34	0,22	-0,18
Schwab & England [%]	72,11	5,35	0,23	0,32
PDQ-39 [score]	44,84	13,53	1,12	1,27

Skewness index values as well as values of kurtosis indicate that the distributions of the majority of the measured data do not deviate from the Gauss-Laplace curve.

To determine the significance of differences of mean values between the experimental and control groups prior to the experiment, a t test for independent samples was used. Before this test had been applied, the compatibility of the distribution of results and the normal distribution was stated and no differences between the variances of all the results obtained in the study groups were found. The results of the t-student test for groups of women and men are shown in Tables 5.1.5. and 5.1.6.

Tab.5.1.5. Comparison of the results obtained by the experimental (EW) and control (CW) group of women prior to the experiment.

Variable		EW		CW		Relative difference	Absolute difference	T test values	
		$\bar{x}1$	S	$\bar{x}2$	S	$\bar{x}1-\bar{x}2$	$\bar{x}1-\bar{x}2(\%)$	T	p
Age [y]		71,23	5,89	70,36	7,15	0,87	1,22	0,33	0,75
Period of illness [y]		6,62	2,26	6,09	2,02	0,52	7,93	0,59	0,56
UPDRS	part I [score]	3,00	1,68	2,91	1,58	0,09	3,03	-1,81	0,17
	part II [score]	15,38	7,76	15,91	4,44	-0,52	-3,41	-1,13	0,28
	part III[score]	22,00	9,35	22,00	5,10	0,00	0,00	0,55	-0,62
	part I, II, III [score]	40,38	16,99	40,82	9,16	-0,43	-1,07	-0,93	0,37
Schwab & England [%]		72,31	5,99	73,64	5,05	-1,33	-1,84	1,00	0,00
PDQ-39 [score]		39,00	20,44	41,45	14,16	-2,45	-6,29	-1,01	0,34

$\bar{x}1$ – mean of the studied parameters in the experimental group,,
$\bar{x}2$ – mean of the studied parameters in the control group,,
S – standard deviation,
t – t-student test value,
p – degree of probability.

Absolute differences between the control and experimental groups of women during the course of the disease (7.93%) and the results of PDQ-39 test (-6.29%) as a result of the t-student test are not statistically significant.

Tab.5.1.6. Comparison of the results obtained by the experimental (EM) and control (CM) group of men prior to the experiment.

Variable		EM		CM		Relative difference	Absolute difference	T test value	
		$\bar{x}1$	S	$\bar{x}2$	S	$\bar{x}1-\bar{x}2$	$\bar{x}1-\bar{x}2(\%)$	T	P
Age [y]		69,70	5,73	70,11	4,20	-0,40	-0,58	-0,26	0,80
Period of illness [y]		8,70	3,69	8,05	2,01	0,65	7,48	0,70	0,49
UPDRS	part I [score]	2,41	1,15	2,26	1,05	0,14	5,99	0.43	0,67
	part II [score]	15,48	6,01	15,95	5,45	-0,47	-3,01	-0,27	0,79
	part III[score]	21,44	7,00	21,95	6,49	-0,50	-2,35	-0,25	0,81
	part I, II, III [score]	39,33	12,96	40,16	10,34	-0,82	-2,10	-0,23	0,82
Schwab 7 England [%]		72,22	7,51	72,11	5,35	0,12	0,16	0,06	0,95
PDQ-39 [score]		40,52	11,47	44,84	13,53	-4,32	-10,67	-1,17	0,25

$\bar{x}1$ – mean of the studied parameters in the experimental group,
$\bar{x}2$ – mean of the studied parameters in the control group,
S – standard deviation,
t – t-student test value,
p – degree of probability.

Similar as in group of women, absolute difference between the control and the experimental group of men during the course of the disease (7.48%) and the results of the PDQ-39 test (-10.67%) was stated. In all the parameters studied, the differences were not statistically significant.

2. Effect of the rehabilitation on efficiency in performing daily activities

To determine the effect of rehabilitation on the performance of daily activities the analysis of variance for repeated measurements was applied.

Women

In the group of women in the results of all tests, there occurred statistically significant differences between groups. The results of analysis of variance are shown in Table 5.2.1.

Tab. 5.2.1. The results of analysis of variance for repeated measurements in the studied groups of women.

Variable	F	p
UPDRS Part I	9,05	0,006
UPDRS Part I*Group	16,41	0,001
UPDRS Part II	16,02	0,001
UPDRS Part II*Group	41,98	0,000
UPDRS Part III	12,97	0,002
UPDRS Part III*Group	45,73	0,000
UPDRS (I, II, III)	29,07	0,000
UPDRS (I, II, III)*Group	86,45	0,000
Schwab England	8,35	0,009
Schwab England*Group	14,16	0,001
PDQ-39	24,73	0,000
PDQ-39*Group	108,24	0,000

Significant difference when $p < 0.01$

To determine the differences between groups post-hoc tests were applied. The results are shown in Tab. 5.2.2.

Tab.5.2.2. The significance of differences before and after the experiment in the studied groups of women.

Variable	EW			CW		
	$\bar{x}$	S	p	$\bar{x}$	S	p
UPDRS part I Prior EXP [score]	3,00	1,68	0,0004	2,91	1,60	0,898
UPDRS part I Post EXP [score]	2,38	1,71		3,00	1,70	
UPDRS part II Prior EXP [score]	15,38	7,76	0,001	15,90	4,40	0,344
UPDRS part II Post EXP [score]	11,54	6,24		16,80	4,50	
UPDRS part III Prior EXP [score]	22,00	9,35	0,0001	22,00	5,10	0,158
UPDRS part III Post EXP [score]	17,23	8,02		23,50	5,40	
UPDRS (I, II, III) Prior EXP [score]	40,38	16,99	0,0001	40,80	9,20	0,584
UPDRS (I, II, III) Post EXP [score]	31,15	14,41		43,30	9,70	
Schwab & England Prior EXP [%]	72,31	5,99	0,0002	73,60	5,00	0,934
Schwab & England Post EXP [%]	79,23	6,41		72,70	7,90	
PDQ-39 Prior EXP [score]	39,00	20,44	0,0001	41,50	14,20	0,006
PDQ-39 Post EXP [score]	32,31	18,52		43,80	14,60	

Significant difference before and after the experiment (p <0.01)

The results of post-hoc tests revealed a statistically significant difference in test results obtained in the experimental group of women before and after the experiment. In contrast, in the control group was observed only statistically significant difference in the results of PDQ-39 test. It should be noted that the difference in the results in this test was due to enlargement of scores, while the difference in the results in the experimental group was due to the reduction of scores.

Tab.5.2.3. Comparison of the results obtained in the tests conducted before and after the experiment in the study of experimental group of women.

Variable		EW prior		EW post		Relative difference	Absolute difference	post-hoc test
		$\bar{x}_1$	S	$\bar{x}_2$	S	$\bar{x}_1 - \bar{x}_2$	$\bar{x}_1 - \bar{x}_2 (\%)$	p
UPDRS	part I [score]	3,00	1,68	2,38	1,71	0,62	-20,67	0,0003
	part II [score]	15,38	7,76	11,54	6,24	3,84	-24,99	0,0002
	part III [score]	22,00	9,35	17,23	8,02	4,77	-21,68	0,0002
	part I, II, III [score]	40,38	16,99	31,15	14,41	9,23	-22,87	0,0002
Schwab & England [%]		72,31	5,99	79,23	6,41	-6,92	9,57	0,0005
PDQ-39 [score]		39,00	20,44	32,31	18,52	6,69	-17,15	0,0002

Tab.5.2.4. Comparison of the results obtained in the tests conducted before and after the experiment in the study of the control group of women.

Variable		CW prior		CW post		Relative difference	Absolute difference	post-hoc test
		$\bar{x}1$	S	$\bar{x}2$	S	$\bar{x}1-\bar{x}2$	$\bar{x}1-\bar{x}2(\%)$	p
UPDRS	part I [score]	2,91	1,58	3,00	1,67	0,09	3,13	0,8928
	part II [score]	15,91	4,44	16,82	4,53	-0,91	5,71	0,3560
	part III[score]	22,00	5,10	23,45	5,45	-1,45	6,61	0,1697
	part I, II, III [score]	40,82	9,16	43,27	9,67	-2,45	6,01	0,0646
Schwab & England [%]		73,64	5,05	72,73	7,86	0,91	-1,23	0,9331
PDQ-39 [score]		41,45	14,16	43,82	14,59	-2,36	5,70	**0,0066**

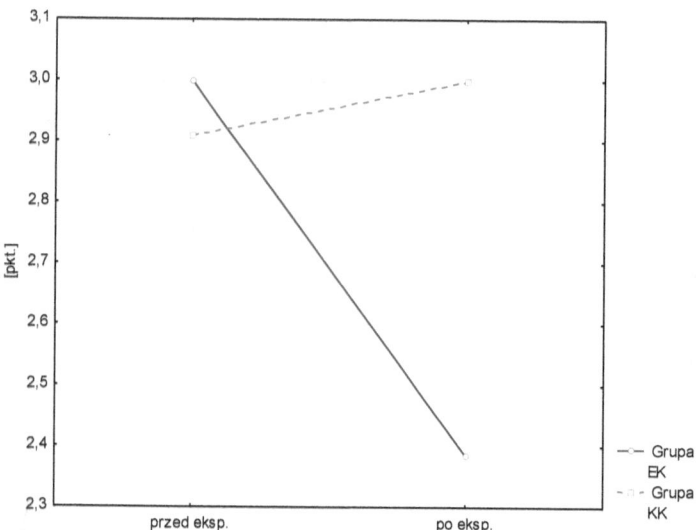

Fig.5.2.1. The results of Part I of the UPDRS test before and after the experiment.

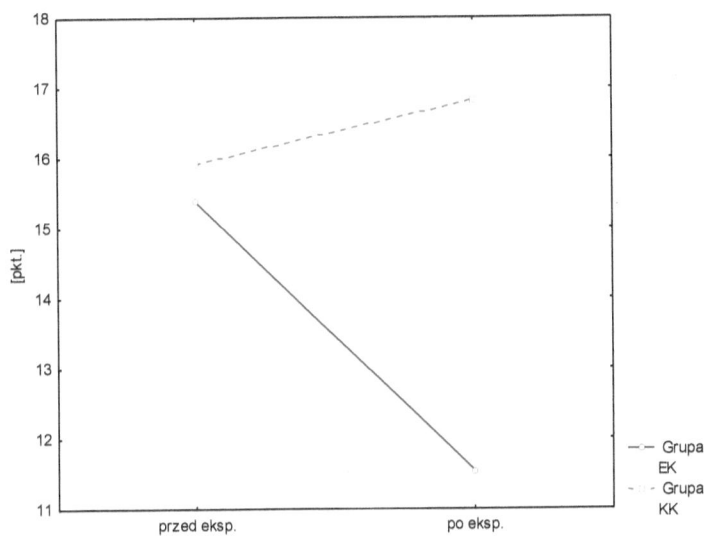

Fig.5.2.2. The results of Part II of the UPDRS test before and after the experiment.

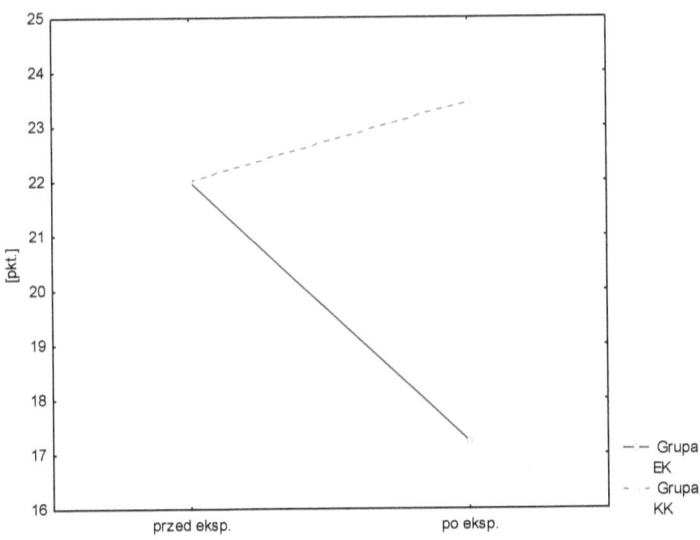

Fig.5.2.3. The results of Part III of the UPDRS test before and after the experiment.

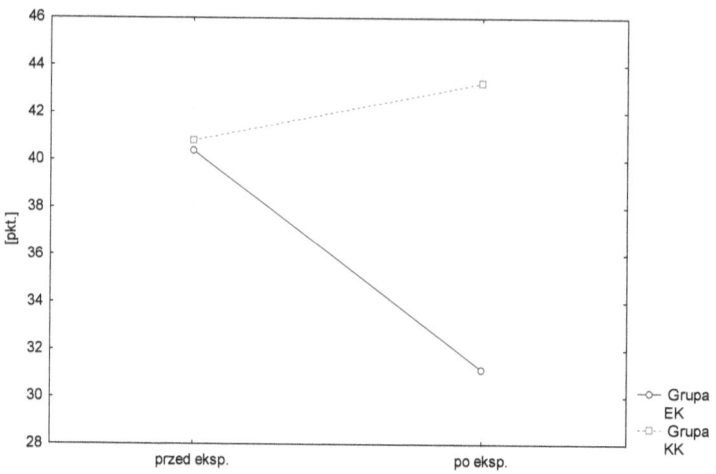

Fig.5.2.4. The results of the UPDRS test (I, II, III) before and after the experiment.

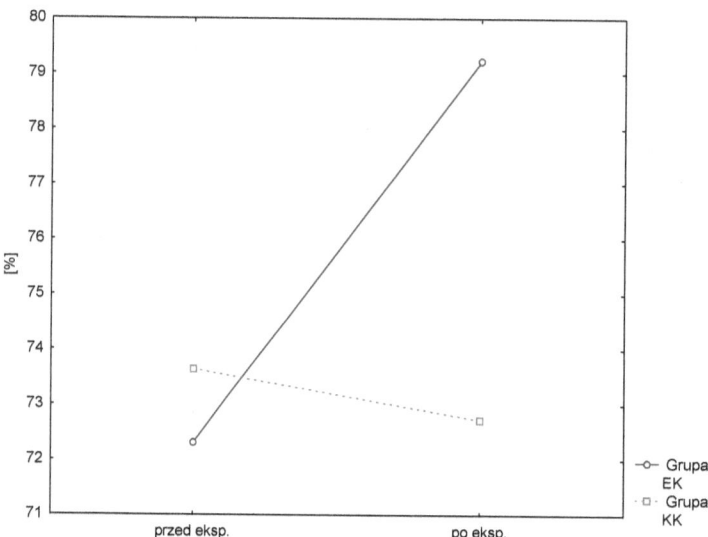

Fig.5.2.5. The results of the Schwab and England test before and after the experiment.

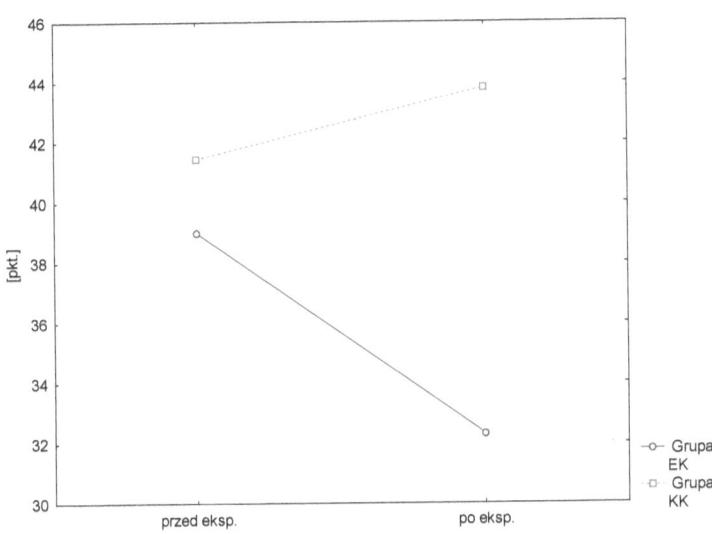

Fig.5.2.6. The results of the PDQ-39 test before and after the experiment.

Men

The analysis of variance showed a statistically significant difference between the groups of men before and after the experiment in any of the tests. The results of the analysis of variance are shown in Table. 5.2.5.

Tab. 5.2.5. The results of analysis of variance for repeated measurements in studied groups of men.

Variable	F	p
UPDRS Part I	3,42	0,071
UPDRS Part I*Group	11,01	0,002
UPDRS PartII	2,05	0,159
UPDRS Part II*Group	66,68	0,000
UPDRS Part III	33,95	0,000
UPDRS Part III*Group	66,67	0,000
UPDRS (I, II, III)	58,66	0,000
UPDRS (I, II, III) *Group	117,24	0,000
Schwab England	11,06	0,002
Schwab England*Group	38,02	0,000
PDQ-39	13,46	0,001
PDQ-39*Group	69,09	0,000

Significant difference when $p < 0.01$

To determine the differences between the groups we used a post-hoc tests. The results are shown in Tab.5.2.6.

Tab.5.2.6. The significance of differences in the studied tests before and after the experiment in the groups of men.

Variable	EM			CM		
	$\bar{x}$	S	P	$\bar{x}$	S	p
UPDRS part I Prior EXP [score]	2,41	1,15	0,0013	2,26	1,05	0,7735
UPDRS part I Post EXP [score]	2,04	1,09		2,37	0,96	
UPDRS part II Prior EXP [score]	15,48	6,01	0,0001	15,95	5,45	0,4482
UPDRS part II Post EXP [score]	12,26	4,84		16,47	5,74	
UPDRS part III Prior EXP [score]	21,44	7,00	0,0001	21,95	6,49	0,4371
UPDRS part III Post EXP [score]	17,67	5,72		22,58	6,76	
UPDRS (I, II, III) Prior EXP [score]	39,33	12,96	0,0001	40,16	10,34	0,1797
UPDRS (I, II, III) Post EXP [score]	31,96	10,71		41,42	10,93	
Schwab & England Prior EXP [%]	72,22	7,51	0,0001	72,11	5,35	0,2629
Schwab & England Post EXP [%]	79,26	5,50		70,00	7,45	
PDQ-39 Prior EXP [score]	40,52	11,47	0,0001	44,84	13,53	0,0206
PDQ-39 Post Exp [score]	33,59	8,97		47,53	13,35	

Significance of differences before and after the experiment when p <0.01

Tab.5.2.7. Comparison of the results obtained in the tests conducted before and after the experiment in the studied experimental group of men.

Variable		EM prior		EM post		Relative difference	Absolute difference	post-hoc test
		$\bar{x}1$	S	$\bar{x}2$	S	$\bar{x}1-\bar{x}2$	$\bar{x}1-\bar{x}2(\%)$	p
UPDRS	Part I [score]	2,41	1,15	2,04	1,09	0,37	-15,38	0,0014
	Part II [score]	15,48	6,01	12,26	4,84	3,22	-20,81	0,0002
	Part III [score]	21,44	7,00	17,67	5,72	3,78	-17,62	0,0002
	Part I, II, III [score]	39,33	12,96	31,96	10,71	7,37	-18,74	0,0002
Schwab & England [%]		72,22	7,51	79,26	5,50	-7,04	9,74	0,0002
PDQ-39 [score]		40,52	11,47	33,59	8,97	6,93	-17,09	0,0002

Tab.5.2.8. Comparison of the results obtained in the tests conducted before and after the experiment in the studied control group of men.

Variable		CM prior		CM post		Relative difference	Absolute difference	post-hoc test
		$\bar{x}1$	S	$\bar{x}2$	S	$\bar{x}1-\bar{x}2$	$\bar{x}1-\bar{x}2(\%)$	p
UPDRS	Part I [score]	2,26	1,05	2,37	0,96	-0,11	4,65	0,7736
	Part II [score]	15,95	5,45	16,47	5,74	-0,53	3,30	0,4483
	Part III[score]	21,95	6,49	22,58	6,76	-0,63	2,88	0,4307
	Part I, II, III [score]	40,16	10,34	41,42	10,93	-1,26	3,15	0,1798
Schwab & England [%]		72,11	5,35	70,00	7,45	2,11	-2,92	0,2630
PDQ-39 [score]		44,84	13,53	47,53	13,35	-2,68	5,99	**0,0206**

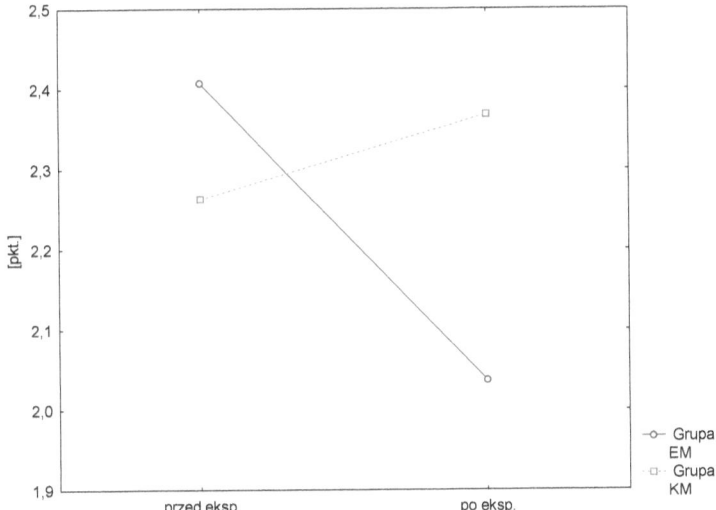

Fig.5.2.7. The results of Part I of the UPDRS test before and after the experiment.

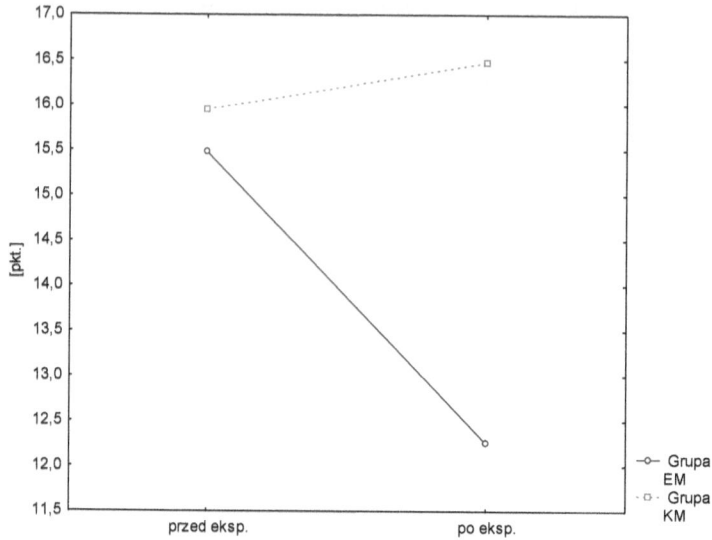

Fig.5.2.8. The results of Part II of the UPDRS test before and after the experiment.

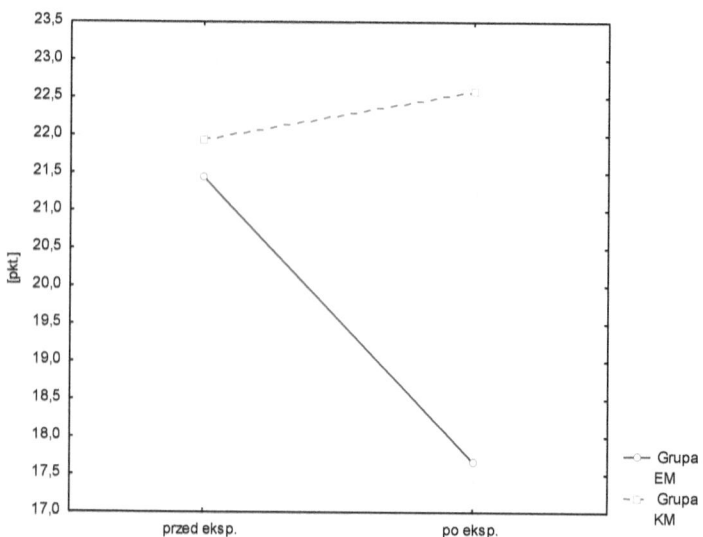

Fig.5.2.9. The results of Part III of the UPDRS test before and after the experiment.

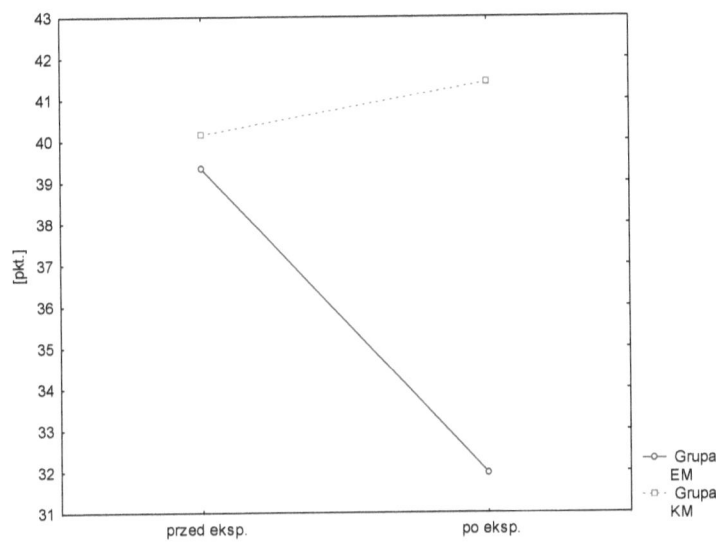

Fig.5.2.10. The results of the UPDRS test (I, II, III) before and after the experiment.

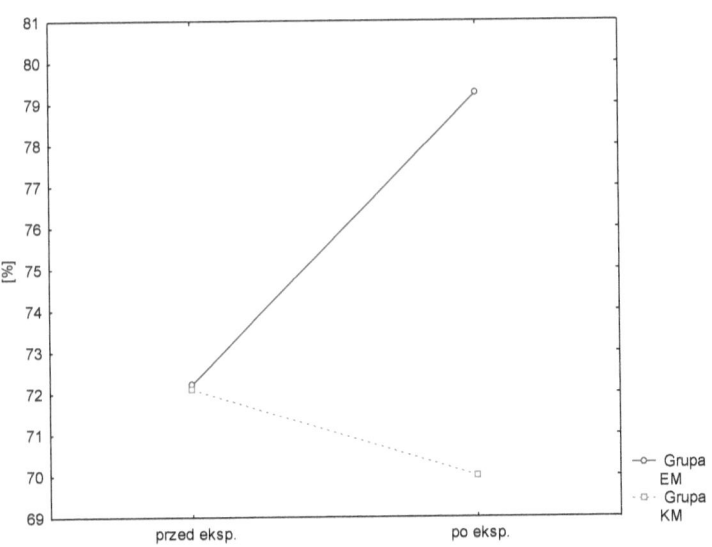

Fig.5.2.11. Test results of the Schwab and England test before and after the experiment.

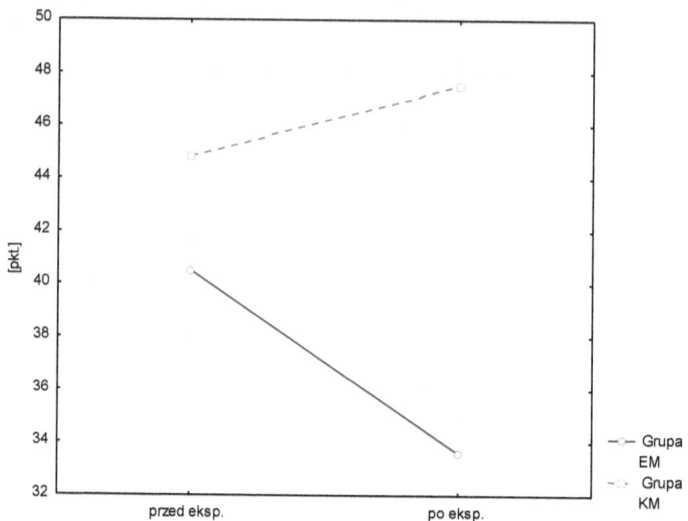

Fig.5.2.12. The results of the PDQ-39 test before and after the experiment.

3. Response of PD patients to exercises depending on the selected factors

In search of factors determining the effectiveness of rehabilitation, the author calculated Spearman's rank correlation coefficients between changes in the efficiency of everyday life as expressed in the results of tests and selected factors: age, period of illness and gender. The results are shown in Tab.5.3.1.

Tab.5.3.1. The values of Spearman's rank correlation coefficients

Group	Vaariables	R
EW	Age & UPDRS I	0,265
	Age & UPDRS II	-0,215
	Age & UPDRS III	-0,387
	Age & UPDRS (I, II, III)	**-0,714**
	Age & Schwab England	-0,517
	Age & PDQ-39	**-0,550**
	Period of illness & UPDRS I	0,444
	Period of illness & UPDRS II	0,337
	Period of illness & UPDRS III	-0,413
	Period of illness & UPDRS (I, II, III)	0,276
	Period of illness & Schwab England	**0,554**
	Period of illness & PDQ-39	**0,590**
EM	Age & UPDRS część I	-0,276
	Age & UPDRS część II	0,169
	Age & UPDRS część III	0,217
	Age & UPDRS (I, II, III)	0,114
	Age & Schwab England	0,343
	Age & PDQ-39	-0,027
	Period of illness & UPDRS I	-0,028
	Period of illness & UPDRS II	-0,115
	Period of illness & UPDRS III	0,166
	Period of illness & UPDRS (I, II, III)	0,017
	Period of illness & Schwab England	**0,683**
	Period of illness & PDQ-39	**-0,520**

Analysis of correlation coefficients showed a high correlation between the effectiveness of rehabilitation measured by the Schwab and England test and PDQ-39 test and the period of illness. This relationship occurred both in the experimental group of women and men.

The highest correlation was observed in the experimental group of men between the results of the UPDRS test and the age. It is a negative correlation which should be interpreted in such a way that with age the effectiveness of rehabilitation measured by the UPDRS test (parts I-III) decreases.

4. Discussion

Commonly there is a conviction of the need for rehabilitation for people with PD. The authors who deal with the disease obtain that the systematic participation in rehabilitation significantly reduces the severity of PD's symptoms and is an essential complement to the medical treatment. Because of the slowly progressive nature of the disease, the form of rehabilitation of this group of patients differs from the rehabilitation in other disease entities. It is easier to maintain the level of functionality than restore functions that were lost as the result of inactivity. This has as a consequence the need for earliness, continuity and systematic rehabilitation.

The results of research carried out in this paper confirmed the thesis of the impact of rehabilitation in the treatment of patients with PD referred to the research of quality of life.

Documented research of the results provide arguments about the applicability of tests to assess quality of life, if a research scope will be set and research methods will be correct. These conditions were complied in this study.

In all the conducted tests, that subjects showed a statistically significant difference before and after the experiment, which included 12 weeks of rehabilitation. The results of analysis of variance both in women and men (Tab.5.2.1., Tab.5.2.5.) indicate statistically significant differences taking into account the factor of division between experimental and control groups, and participation in the experiment. The largest percentage improvement in the experimental group of women occurred in the results of the UPDRS test (22.87%). Physical exercise resulted in improvement in mobility. In next trials tested women obtained smaller score values, which indicates improvement. In the UPDRS test the assessment of performance is made basing on a score scale. 0 point means no change, and 4 points mean the greatest severity of symptoms in a given sample.

It should also be noted that there was a decrease in the efficiency levels in the control group of women, as evidenced by the greater number of points obtained in the test after the experiment (Tab.5.2.2., Fig.5.2.4.). However, the changes were statistically insignificant, so the performance status within three months of the experiment in the control group of women did not change. In relation to a statistically significant improvement of efficiency in the experimental group, leads to the conclusion that physical activity reduces the occurrence of motor symptoms of PD.

Similar results were obtained in the group of men. According to physical testing using the UPDRS method in the experimental group, an improvement of 18.74% was observed, with the largest one in part II (20,81%). The differences were statistically significant. In the control group at the same time there were no statistically significant changes in physical performance.

Analyzing the results of the research attention should be paid to the occurrence of improvement in the experimental groups in all studied parts of the UPDRS i.e. I - assessment of intellectual and mood disorders, II - assessment of activities of daily living, III - study of the musculoskeletal system. Particularly interesting is the improvement of the results in Part I. The experiment performed included fitness classes and functional training, aimed primarily at increasing the range of motion, improve balance, motor skills and walking. The main emphasis was placed on the ability to cope with activities of daily living. There have been no psychological therapy, however, we observed a positive effect of physical activity also on the mental condition. Similar results were obtained by Dam et al. [1996]. Leading physiotherapy classes for 12 months he observed a reduction in the level of depression in the study group. However, the results of other studies did not support these conclusions. Comella et al. [1994] and Nieuwboer et al. [2001] after application of fitness classes found no improvement in mental status in relation to the control group. Similar results were obtained by Katsikitis, Pilowsky [1996] after a 4-week rehabilitation. Authors reported on the impact of fitness classes on mental state are not clear in the case of using only physical activities, but if the therapeutic activities are multidisciplinary then effects also occur in a range of all studied areas. Evidence of this are researches by Trend et al. [2002] and Wade et al. [2002]. For a period of 12 and 6 months leading multidisciplinary therapy comprising: an individual physiotherapy, occupational therapy, speech and language therapy, specialist nursing care, and also support and education, they observed a significant, immediate improvement in a range of all studied areas, but after six months from the end of experiment, the patients had only a slight improvement in mobility. The conclusion was made that there is the need for comprehensive rehabilitation of patients with PD.

In the literature, there are available tests results that assess the efficacy of physical exercise on the severity of the symptoms of PD. These include various forms of activities and a variety of ways to assess its effectiveness [Goodwin et al. 2008, Tomlison et al. 2012]. Mitchell et al. [1987] were leading flexibility classes for a period of eight weeks and he observed a statistically significant improvement in the functional capabilities of patients. However, studies were carried out just on a group of 7 people. The studies conducted by Formisano et al. [1992] conducted a larger group. In the experimental group of 16 persons, physical activities were carried out three times a week for one hour over a period of 4 months. A statistically significant improvement was measured by measuring the characteristics of gait. Walk on time, step length measurement and assessment of posture were measures of the effectiveness of rehabilitation activities conducted by Scandalis et al. [2001]. Classes were conducted at a frequency of 2 times a week for 8 weeks and were mainly aimed at improving gait by walking at a specified rate and training in low mountains. In the group of 14 people they found improvement in the examined parameters. The above studies mainly focused on the assessment of the efficiency of gait and were conducted in small research groups, so a comparison of the results of this research paper is difficult. The paper focuses on the measurement of the efficiency in a wider range.

Evaluating the effectiveness of physical activities using the scale of activities of daily living (ADL) more comprehensively illustrates the changes in the functional capabilities of patients and it is widely used. ADL scale was used by Comell et al. [1994] to evaluate the effectiveness of rehabilitation. In these studies, patients with PD participated in fitness classes 3 times a week for 1 hour over a period of four weeks. The level of efficiency was measured in relation to the comparative group. A significant improvement was observed after the exercise period but after six months without exercises there was no difference between the groups. The level of performance of the experimental group returned to baseline. Similar results were obtained by Nieuwboer et al. [2001]. They obtained results improvement in subjects in ADL scale after 3-month of rehabilitation, however, after discontinuation of classes, after another period of 3 months, there was a return to baseline.

To assess the effects of their research on a group of people with PD Pacchetti et al. [2000] also used the ADL scale. In contrast to the above studies, fitness classes based mainly on music fitness classes, and included the period of three months (from 1.5 to 2 hours per week). Following treatment differences were statistically significant, but remained only for a period of two months.

As described above, the vast majority of studies noticed the improvement in the efficiency after application of physical therapy. In each work, authors obtained an improvement of at least one of the tests elements immediately after the experiments. These included a variety of rehabilitation programs, or only one of its forms. They were carried out in small study groups and not all of them included a control group. In addition, attention was paid mainly to the statistical results, to a lesser extent, paying attention to the size of the clinical changes and that is most relevant for patients. For example, An important element is to improve the efficiency of time walking a certain distance, but only when it is considered in the context of improving the usefulness in everyday life and not to set a new record [Gage, Storey 2004].

In relation to the reports presented in the literature, research in this paper were characterized by a much greater research group, which gives a greater ability to generalize the results. Also characterized by a different approach to physical fitness, which were focused on the ability to perform activities of daily living. This program was adapted to rehabilitation activities and tests that we applied.

In the experimental group of women in Part II of the UPDRS test (evaluation of activities of daily living) a statistically significant improvement of 24.99% was observed, while in the group of men also statistically significant by 20.81%. In Part III of the UPDRS test (the study of motion) an improvement in 21.68% for women, and in 17.62% for men was noticed. Part I, II, III of the UPDRS test allows for the assessment of patients in a point scale in many aspects, while applied study of the Schwab and England scale gives a greater variety of assessment, however, a more global. Also, the measurement of the efficiency of using this scale allowed for the observation of the positive impact of rehabilitation applied to the experimental groups. For women, there was a statistically significant improvement of 9.57% and for men by 9.74%.

These results clearly show the high reactivity of the respondents to the applied physical exercise. Quality of life assessment tests that were applied showed the definite improvement of this quality. This issue is related to a slightly larger aspect of the impact of physical activity on patients bodies. Scientific studies clearly show that an increase in physical activity at an earlier constraint, cause the improvement of physical function, regardless of age. Everyone adapts to the new conditions if they do not exceed the adaptive capacity. For older people physical activity delays the involution. This also applies to people with PD, and the physical activity should be focused on the efficiency of activities of daily living. Literature describes studies that assess the impact of certain measures of "training" on patients with PD. Bergen et al. [2002] used oxygen efforts three times a week for 16 weeks and he obtained the improved of VO_{2max} both in patients with PD, and in healthy subjects in comparison to a group without this kind of practice. Similar results were achieved by Bridgewater, Sharpe [1996, 1998], to obtain an improvement of selected performance parameters of circulatory he used aerobic exercise twice a week for 12 weeks. Increasing fitness achievements supported by sensory techniques of repeats as compared to conventional therapy received Dam et al. [1996], Marchese et al. [2000], Thaut et al. [1996]. The use of osteopathic manipulation resulted in clinical improvement of the walk in researches by Wells et al. [1999]. Improvement of the efficiency was measured by the mobility of the arms and by agility also were obtained after applying the general development of exercise [Behrman et al. 2000, Worringham, Stelmach 1990].

For the evaluation of the results of the experiment described, besides to the objective tests described above, there were used subjective assessment of the quality of life the PDQ-39 test. In both, the experimental groups of men and women was statistically significant improvement in results. For women by 17.15%, while for men by 17.09%. Statistically significant changes have also occurred in control groups. It was, however, a deterioration evaluation. On this basis it can be concluded that the subjective evaluation is also associated with the psychological state of the respondents and the development of the disease. As described in the literature studies in which an attempt was made of using a simultaneous impact of integrated measures on patients with PD, were observed differences in effectiveness. Achieved positive results in terms of both physical and mental. In these studies, the duration of the course of the week classes was different. Gauthier et al. [1987] conducted 20 hours of group occupational therapy, physiotherapy and education during the period of five weeks, while in the experiment by Trend et al. [2002], Wade et al. [2002] classes include 36 hours per week of individual physiotherapy, occupational therapy, speech therapy, nursing care, social care, education and support group for a period of six weeks. In both cases, the achieved sustained therapeutic effects during period after end of experiment (respectively 12 and 6 months).

As described in the literature the studies involving patients with PD, the combination of physical therapy with occupational therapy does not always give positive results. Gibberd et al. [1987] by using a combination of physiotherapy and occupational therapy in eight groups for a period of more than four weeks achieved a statistically insignificant change to maintain independent functioning and independence. In contrast, Fiorani et al. [1997], Toole et al. [2000] led the experiment in which one group was treated only with physiotherapy classes and the other involved both classes of physiotherapy and occupational therapy and they put forward a proposal for a major merger of the two forms of activity to improve the independence and quality of life.

Another aspect of this paper research was to determine the response of patients with PD to exercise depending on the selected factors. The author studied the dependence on sex, age and disease duration. To determine this relationship the correlation coefficient for changes in physical efficiency determined by specific results of tests and selected factors was calculated. Statistical calculations showed no dependence with respect to gender, which is confirmed in the literature. In all the available experiments on the effect of physical exercise on physical fitness, the authors did not differentiate respondents by gender [Gage, Storey 2004].

The biggest dependence occurred in relation to the duration of the disease, which is associated with the severity of lameness. This is confirmed by studies developed by Slawek and Derejko [2002] who found a relationship between disease duration and severity of the factors affecting the quality of life.

The analysis of the literature and the results obtained in this paper suggest that further research on the effectiveness of rehabilitation in patients with PD, most likely will have to focus on multidisciplinary activities. The interaction of specialists from different fields can give an opportunity to understand the impact of various components improving the body of patients and understand their interaction. Some studies showed the positive impact of merger physiotherapy, occupational therapy and speech therapy on psychological well-being, as an additional effect post experimental. However, in some studies [Comella et al. 1994, Nieuwboer et al., 2001] there was no influence at all. The vast majority of studies reported in the literature indicate a positive effect on the efficiency of the physical activities of patients, which, however, decreases with time, indicating a need to run rehabilitation in a systematic way. The improvement of emotional well-being may also be important effect of "placebo" of the treatment, as shown in studies that included control groups. With rehabilitation patients can extend the ability to function normally. The beginning of physical therapy in the early stage of the disease can significantly delay its progress and especially senility. It seems necessary to collect data that may help in coping with Parkinson's disease, because with the aging of population the number of patients with Parkinson's disease will certainly grow.

5. Conclusions

The research on the impact of rehabilitation on the severity of motor symptoms carried out in the paper allows the author to draw the following conclusions:

1. As a result of systematic rehabilitation of patients with Parkinson's disease the improvement of the efficiency or lack of severity of symptoms compared with patients who did not participate in rehabilitation activities was achieved.

2. In patients with Parkinson's disease by systematically pursued rehabilitation improvements in daily activities and quality of life were achieved.

3. There was no difference in terms of the improvement in efficiency due to gender.

4. The duration of the disease and the age of the patients were negative factors in relation to the improvement of efficiency despite the use of rehabilitation.

The study made it possible to verify the research hypothesis:

Systematically conducted rehabilitation reduces the consequences of Parkinson's disease, allows for improvement in daily activities. The use of physical rehabilitation improves the quality of life of patients with Parkinson's disease.

Reference

1. Azulay J.P., Mesure S., Amblard B., Blin O., Sangla I., Pouget J.(1999): Visual control of locomotion in Parkinson's disease. Brain, 122:111-120.
2. Babinski J., Jarkowski B., Plichet V.(1921): Kinesie paradoxale: mutisme Parkinsonie. Revue Neurologique, 37:1266-1270.
3. Banks M., Caird F.(1989): Physiotherapy benefits with Parkinson's disease. Clinical Rehabilitation, 3:11-16.
4. Banks P., Lawrence M. (2006): The Disability Discrimination Act, a necessary, but not sufficient safeguard for people with progressive conditions in the workplace? The experiences of younger people with Parkinson's disease. Disability and Rehabilitation, 28(1):13-24.
5. Beattie A., Caird F.I.(1980): The occupational therapist and the patient with Parkinson's disease. British Medical Journal, 280:1354-55.
6. Beckley D.J., Bloem B.R., Van Dijk J.G., Roos R.A.C., Remler M.P.(1991): Electrophysiological corelates of postura instability in Parkinson,s disease. Electroencephalography and Clinical Neurophysiology, 81:263-268.
7. Behrman A., Teitelbaum P., Cauraugh J.H.(1998): Verbal instructional sets to normalise the temporal and spatial gait variables in Parkinson's disease. Journal of Neurology, Neurosurgery and Psychiatry, 65:580-582.
8. Behrman A.L., Cauraugh J.H., Light K.E.(2000): Practice as an intervention to improve speeded motor performance and motor learning in Parkinson's disease. Journal of the Neurological Sciences, 174:127-36.
9. Benecke R., Rothwell J.C., Dick J.P., Day B.L., Marsden C.D.(1987): Disturbance of sequential movements in patients with Parkinson's disease. Journal of Neurology, 110(2):361-379.
10. Bergen J., Toole T., Elliott R., Wallace B., Robinson K., Maitland C.(2002): Aerobic exercise intervention improves aerobic capacity and movement initiation in Parkinson's disease patients. Neurorehabilitation, 17:161-68.
11. Biggins C.A., Boyd J.L., Harrop F.M., Madeley P., Mindham R.H., Randall J.I., Spokes E.G.(1992): A controlled, longitudinal study of dementia in Parkinson's disease. Journal of Neurology, Neurosurgery and Psychiatry, 55:566-571.
12. Błaszczyk J.W., Hansen P.D., Lowe D.L.(1993): Evaluation of the postural stability in man: movement and posture interaction. Acta Neurobiologiae Experimentalis, 53(1):155-160.
13. Błaszczyk J.W., Orawiec R., Duda-Kłodowska D., Opala G.(2007): Assessment of postural instability in patients with Parkinson's disease. Experimental Brain Research, 183(1):107-14.
14. Bond J., Morris M.E.(2000): Goal-directed secondary motor tasks: their effects on gait in subjects with Parkinson disease. Archives of Physical Medicine and Rehabilitation, 81:110-16.
15. Borrione P, Tranchita E, Sansone P, Parisi A.(2014): Effects of physical activity in Parkinson's disease: A new tool for rehabilitation. World Journal of Methodology, 26,4(3):133-143.

16. Brauer S.G., Morris M.E.(2010): Can people with Parkinson's disease improve dual tasking when walking? Gait Posture, 31:229-233.
17. Bridgewater K., Sharpe M.(1996): Aerobic exercise and early Parkinson's disease. Neurorehabilitation and Neural Repair, 10(4):233-241.
18. Bridgewater K., Sharpe M.(1998): Trunk muscle training in early Parkinson's disease. Physical Therapy, 78(6):566-577.
19. Brusse K., Zimdars S., Zalewski K., Steffen T.(2005): Testing functional performance in people with Parkinson disease. Physical Therapy, 2:134-141.
20. Calne S.M., Lidstone S.C., Kumar A.(2008): Psychosocial issues in young-onset Parkinson's disease: current research and challenges. Parkinsonism and Related Disorders, 14(2):143-50.
21. Canning C.G., Ada L., Woodhouse E.(2008): Multiple-task walking training in people with mild to moderate Parkinson's disease: a pilot study. Clinical Rehabilitation, 22:226-33.
22. Carter J.(1995): Exercise. [In:] Johnson A., [ed.]:Young Parkinson,s handbook. New York, American Parkinson Disease Association, 29-33.
23. Carter J.H., Stewart B.J., Archbold P.G., Inoue I., Jaglin J., Lannon M., Rost-Ruffner E., Tennis M., McDermott M.P., Amyot D., Barter R., Cornelius L., Demong C., Dobson J., Duff J., Erickson J., Gardiner N., Gauger L., Gray P., Kanigan B., Kiryluk B., Lewis P., Mistura K., Malapira T., Zoog K.(1998): Living with a person who has Parkinson's disease: the spouse's perspective by stage of disease. Parkinson's Study Group. Movement Disorders, 13(1): 20-28.
24. Chalimoniuk M., Langford J.(2007): The effect of a subchronic, intermittet L-DOPA treatment on nNOS and sCG expression and activity in the striatum and midbrain of normal and MPTP-treated mice. Neurochemistry International, 50(6):821-833.
25. Cholewa J, Boczarska-Jedynak M, Opala G.(2013): Influence of physiotherapy on severity of motor symptoms and quality of life in patients with Parkinson disease. Neurologia i Neurochirurgia Polska, 47(3):256-262.
26. Cholewa J.:(2014): Rehabilitation Procedures Aimed at Decreasing Motor Symptoms in Parkinson's Disease. International Journal of Physical Medicine and Rehabilitation, S5:009. doi: 10.4172/2329-9096.S5-009.
27. Comella C.L., Stebbins G., Brown-Toms N., Goetz C.(1994): Physical therapy and Parkinson's disease: A controlled clinical trial. Neurology, 44:376-78.
28. Crow R., Gage H., Hart S., Hampson S., Kimber A., Thomas H.(1999): Role of expectancies in the placebo effect and their use in the delivery of health care. Health Technology Assessment, 3(3):1-96.
29. Dam M., Tonin P., Casson S., Bracco F., Piron L., Pizzolato G., Battistin L.(1996): Effects of conventional and sensory enhanced physiotherapy on disability in Parkinson's disease patients. Advances in Neurology, 69:551-555.
30. Deane KH, Jones D, Ellis-Hill C. Clarke CE, Playford ED, Ben-Shlomo Y. (2001): A comparison of physiotherapy techniques for patients with Parkinson's disease. The Cochrane database of systematic reviews, CD 002815.

31. del Olmo MF, Cudeiro J.(2005): Temporal variability of gait in Parkinson disease: effects of a rehabilitation programme based on rhythmic sound cues. Parkinsonism and Related Disorders, 11:25-33.
32. Diamond S.G., Markham C.H., Hoehn M.M., NcDowell F.H., Muenter M.D.(1990): An examination of male-female differences in progression and mortality of Parkinson's disease. Neurology, 40(5):763-766.
33. Etherington D., Ingold J.(2012): Welfare to work and the inclusive labour market: a comparative study of activation policies for disability and long-term sickness benefit claimants in the UK and Denmark. Journal of European social Policy, 22(1):30-44.
34. Fahn S., Elton R.(1987): Unified Parkinson's disease rating scale. [In:] Fahn S, Marsden CD, Goldstein M, Calne DB, editors. Recent developments in Parkinson's disease. New York: MacMillan; p 153-63.
35. Falvo M.J., Schilling B.K., Earhart G.M.(2008): Parkinson's Disease and Resistive Exercise: Rationale, Review and Recommendations. Movement Disorders, 23(1): 1-11.
36. Fiorani C., Mari R., Bartolini M., Ceravolo M., Provinciali L.(1997): Occupational therapy increases ADL and quality of life in Parkinsonism patients. Rehabilitation and Physiotherapy, 12:134-35.
37. Formisano R., Pratesi L., Modarelli F., Bonifati V., Meco G.(1992): Rehabilitation and Parkinson's disease. Scandinavian Journal of Rehabilitation Medicine, 24(3):157-60.
38. Foti D.J., Cummings J.L.(1997) Neurobehavioral aspects of movement disorders. [W:] Watts R.L., Koller W.C.[ed.] Movement disorders. Neurologic principles and practice. New York: McGraw-Hill, 15-30.
39. Frazzitta G., Maestri R., Uccellini D., Bertotti G., Abelli P.(2009): Rehabilitation treatment of gait in patients with Parkinson's disease with freezing: a comparison between two physical therapy protocols using visual and auditory cues with or without treadmill training. Movement Disorders, 24:1139-1143.
40. Friedman A., Bauminger E., Gałązka-Friedman J.(1996): Is iron involved in the pathogenesis of Parkinson's disease – Mossbauer spectroscopy study of substantia nigra in control and disease brians. Neurologia and Neurochirurgia Polska, 30(supl.2):95-103.
41. Friedman A.(1994): Old-onset Parkinson's disease compared with young-onset disease: clinical differences and similarities. Acta Neurologica Scandinavica, 89(4):258-261.
42. Friedman A., Barcikowska M.(1994): Dementia in Parkinson's disease. Dementia, 5(1):12-16.
43. Gage H., Storey L.(2004): Rehabilitation for Parkinson's disease: a systematic review of available evidence. Clinical Rehabilitation, 18:463-482.
44. Galletly R., Brauer S.G.(2005): Does the type of concurrent task affect preferred and cued gait in people with Parkinson's disease? Australian Journal of Physiotherapy, 51:175–80.

45. Gauthier L., Dalziel S., Gauthier S.(1987): The benefits of group occupational therapy for patients with Parkinson's disease. American Journal of Occupational Therapy, 41:360-365.
46. Gibberd F.B., Page N.G., Spencer K.M., Kinnear E., Hawksworth J.B.(1981): Controlled trial of physiotherapy and occupational therapy for Parkinson's disease. British Medical Journal, 282:1196.
47. Gleb D.J., Oliver E., Gilman S.(1999): Diagnostic criteria for Parkinson's disease. Archives of Neurology, 56:3-9.
48. Goebel S., Atanassov L., Köhnken G., Mehdorn H.M., Leplow B. (2013): Understanding quantitative and qualitative figural fluency in patients with Parkinson's disease. Neurology Science, 34(8): 1383-1390.
49. Goetz C., Stebbins G.T., Shale H.M., Lang A.E., Chernik D.A., Chmura T.A., Ahlskog J.E., Dorflinger E.E.(1994): Utility of an objective dyskinesia rating scale for Parkinson's disease: inter- and intrarater reliability assessment. Movement Disorders, 9:390-394.
50. Golbe L.(1998): Epidemiology of movement disorders. [In:] Jankowic J., Tolosa E, [ed.] Parkinson,s disease and movement disorders. Thirds ed., Lippincott Williams and Wilkinns, Baltimore, 119-132.
51. Goodwin V.A., Richards S.H., Taylor R.C., Taylor A.H., Campbell J.L.(2008): The effectiveness of exercise interventions for people with Parkinson's disease: A systematic review and meta-analysis. Movement Disorders, 23(5):631-640.
52. Gueye L., Viallet F., Legallet E., Trouche E.(1998): The use of advance information for motor preparation in Parkinson's disease: effects of cueing and compatibility between warning and imperative stimuli. Brain and Cognition, 38:66-86.
53. Guide to Physical Therapist Practice. (1997), Physical Therapy, 77(11):1160-1656.
54. Herlofson K., Lie S.A., Arsland D., Larsen J.P.(2004): Mortality and Parkinson disease: A community based study. Neurology, 62(2):937-942.
55. Hirsch M.A., Toole T., Maitland C.G., Rider R.A.(2003): The effects of balance training and high-intensity resistance training on persons with idiopathic Parkinson's disease. Archives of Physical Medicine and Rehabilitation, 84 (8):1109-1117.
56. Hoehn M.M., Yahr M.D.(1967): Parkinsonism: onset, progression and mortality. Neurology, 17(5):427-442.
57. Holbrook M., Skilbeck C.E.(1983): An activities index for use with stroke patients. Age Ageing, 12(2):166-170.
58. Howe T.E., Lovgreen B., Cody F.W., Ashton V.J., Oldham J.A.(2003): Auditory cues can modify the gait of persons with early-stage Parkinson's disease: a method for enhancing parkinsonian walking performance? Clinical Rehabilitation, 17:363-367.
59. Hurwitz A.(1989): The benefit of a home exercise regimen for ambulatory Parkinson's disease patients. Journal of Neuroscience Nursing, 21(3):180-184.

60. Iasek R., Bradshowj., Philips J.(1995): Interaction of the basal Anglia and supplementatarymotor area in the elaboration of movement. [W:] Glencross D., Piek J. [ed.] Motor Control and Sensomotor Integration. Amsterdam, the Netherlands, Elsevier, 37-59.
61. Jayasekar R.(2013): Does Physiotherapy Improve the Functional Ability of Patients with Parkinson's Disease? The American Journal of Nursing, 113(2):65-65.
62. Jellinger K.A.(2003): Age-associated prevalence and risk factors of Lewy body pathology in a general population. Acta Neuropathologica, 106(4): 383-384.
63. Jenkinson C., Heffernan C., Doll H., Fitzpatrick R.(2006): The Parkinson's Disease Questionnaire (PDQ-39): evidence for a method of imputing missing data. Age Ageing, 35(5):497-502.
64. Jenkison C., Fitzpatrick R., Peto V.(1997): The Parkinson,s disease questionnaire: user manual for the PDQ-39 – 39, PDQ-39 – 8 and PDQ-39 summary index, heath services research unit, University of Oxford.
65. Kamsma Y., Brouwer W., Lakke J.(1995): Training of compensational strategies for impaired gross motor skills in Parkinson' disease. Physiotherapy Theory and Practice, 11(4):209-229.
66. Karlsen K., Larsen J., Tandberg E., Maeland J.G.(1999): Influence of clinical and demographic variables on quality of life in patients with Parkinson's disease. Journal of Neurology, Neurosurgery and Psychiatry, 66(4): 431-435.
67. Karnofsky D.A., Burchenal J.H.(1949): The clinical evaluation of chemotherapeutic agents in cancer. [In:] Mac Leo C.M., Evaluation of chemotherapeutic agents.(1992), WHO, Quality of Life, Special report, New York.
68. Katsikitis M., Pilowsky J.(1996): A controlled study of facial mobility treatment in Parkinson's disease. Journal of Psychosomatic Research, 40(4):387-396.
69. Katz S., Ford A.B., Moskowitz R.W., Jackson B.A., Jaffe M.W.(1963): Studies of illness in the aged. The Index of ADL: a standardized measure of biological and psychosocial function. Journal of The American Medical Association, 185: 914-919.
70. Keus S.H., Bloem B.R., Hendriks E.J., Bredero-Cohen A.B., Munneke M.(2007): Evidence-based analysis of physical therapy in Parkinson's disease with recommendations for practice and research. Movement Disorders, 22:451-460.
71. Kikuchi E.(1993): Daily living abilities and work abilities of people with Parkinson's disease. Work., 13(3):239-248.
72. Knoke D., Taylor A.E., Saint-Cyr J.A.(1998): The differential effects of cueing on recall in Parkinson's disease and normal subjects. Brain and Cognition, 38:261-74.
73. Knuttson E., Martenson A.(1986): Posture and gait in parkinsonian patients. [In:] Bles W., Brandt T.H.[ed.] Disorders of posture and gait. Elsevier, Amsterdam, New York, 217-229.

74. Koch L., Rumrill P., Conyers L., Wohlford S.(2013): A narriative literature review regarding job retention strategies for people with chronic illnesses. Work:46(1):125-134.
75. Koike Y., Takahashi A.(1997): Autonomic dysfunction in Parkinson's disease. European Neurology, 38(supl.): 8-12.
76. Korchounov A., Bogomazov G.(2006): Employment, medical absenteeism, and disability perception in Parkinson's disease: A pilot double-blind, randomized, placebo-controlled study of entacapone adjunctive therapy. Movement Disorders, 21(12):2220-2224.
77. Kowal S.L., Dall T.M., Chakrabarti R., Storm M.V., Jain A.(2013): The current and projected economic burden of Parkinson's disease in the United States. Movement Disorders, 28(3):311-8.
78. Kritikos A., Leahy C., Bradshaw J.L., Iansek R., Phillips J.G., Bradshaw J.A.(1995): Contingent and non-contingent auditory cueing in Parkinson's disease. Neuropsychologia, 33:1193-203.
79. Kuhn W., Muller T.(1997): Therapie des Morbus Parkinson. Teil 1: Standardtherapie motorischer und nicht motorischer Symptome. Fortschritte Der Neurologie-Psychiatrie, 65(8): 361-375.
80. Lang A.E., Lozano A.M.(1998): Parkinson's disease; first of two parts. The New England Journal of Medicine, 339:1044-1053.
81. Lewis G., Byblow W.D., Walt S.(2000): Stride length regulation in Parkinson's disease: the use of extrinsic, visual cues. Brain, 123:2077-90.
82. Lim I, van Wegen E, de Goede C, Deutekom M., Nieuwboer A., Willems A., Jones D., Rochester L., Kwakkel G.(2005): Effects of external rhythmical cueing on gait in patients with PD: a systematic review. Clinical Rehabilitation, 19:696-713.
83. Litvan I., Bhatia K.P., Burn D.J., Goetz C.G., Lang A.E., McKeith I., Quinn N., Sethi K.D., Shults C., Wenning G.K.(2003): SIC Task Force appraisal of clinical diagnostic criteria for parkinsonian disorders. Movement Disorders, 18: 467-486.
84. Louis E.D., Levy G., Cote L.J., Mejia H., Fahn S., Marder K.(2001): Clinical correlates of Action Tremor in Parkinson's Disease. Archives of Neurology, 58:1630-1634.
85. Majsak M.J., Kamiński T., Gentile A.M., Flanagan J.R.(1998): The reaching movements of patients with Parkinson's disease under self-determined maximal speed and visually cued conditions. British Medical Journal, 121(4):1161-81.
86. Marchese R., Diverio M., Zucchi F., Lentino C., Abbruzzese G.(2000): The role of sensory cues in the rehabilitation of parkinsonian patients: a comparison of two physical therapy protocols.. Movement Disorders, 15(5): 879-883.
87. Martikainen K.K., Luukkaala T.H., Marttila R.J.(2006): Parkinson's disease and working capacity. Movement Disorders, 21(12):2187-2191.
88. Martin J.P.(1967): The Basal Ganglia and Posture. London, England, Pitman Medical.

89. McIntosh G., Brown S.H., Rice R.R., Thaut M.H.(1997): Rhythmic auditorymotor facilitation of gait patterns in patients with Parkinson's disease. Journal of Neurology, Neurosurgery and Psychiatry, 62:22-6.
90. Mitchell P.H., Mertz M.A., Catanzaro M.L.(1987): Group exercise: a nursing therapy in Parkinson's disease. Rehabilitation Nursing, 12(7):242-245.
91. Montgomery J., Erwin B.(2004): Rehabilitative approaches to Parkinson's disease. Parkinsonism and Related Disorders, 10(supl.1), 43.
92. Morris M., Iansek R.(1997): Gait disorders in Parkinson's disease; a framework for physical therapy practice. Neurology Report, 21:125-131.
93. Morris M., Iansek R., Matyas T.A., Summers J.J.(1995): Motor control consideration for gait rehabilitation in Parkinson's disease. [In:] Glencross D., Pick J.(ed.), Motor Control and Sensorimotor Integration. Amsterdam, the Netherlands, Elsevier, 61-93.
94. Morris M.E.(2000): Movement disorders in people with Parkinson disease: a model for physical therapy. Physical Therapy, 80(6):578-597.
95. Morris M.E., Bruce M., Smithson F.(1997): Physiotherapy strategies for people with Parkinson's disease [In:] Morris M.E., Iansek R.(ed.) Parkinson's Disease: A Team Approach. Blacburn, Australia, Busombe-Vicprint, 27-64.
96. Morris M.E., Colier J., Matyas T.A.(1998): Evidence for motor skill learning in Parkinson's disease. [In:] Piek J.(ed.) Motor Behavior and Human Skill, Champaign, III: Human Kinetics Inc, 329-54.
97. Morris M.E., Iansek R., Churchyard A.(1998): The role of the physiotherapist in quantifying movement fluctuations in Parkinson's disease. Australian Journal of Physiotherapy, 44 (2):105-114.
98. Morris M.E., Iansek R., Matyas T.A., Summers J.J.(1994): The pathogenesis of gait hypokinesia in Parkinson's disease. British Medical Journal, 117(5):1169-1181.
99. Morris M.E., Iansek R., Matyas T.A., Summers J.J.(1994): Ability to modulate walking cadence remains intact in Parkinson's disease. Journal of Neurology, Neurosurgery and Psychiatry, 57(12):1532-4.
100. Morris M.E., Iansek R., Matyas T.A., Summers J.J.(1996): Stride length regulation in Parkinson's disease normalization strategies and underlying mechanisms. British Medical Journal, 119(2):551-68.
101. Morris M.E., Iansek R., Matyas T.A., Summers J.L.(1994): The pathogenesis of gait hypokinesia in Parkinson's disease. Brain, 117:1169-1181.
102. Morris M.E.(2000): Movement disorders in people with Parkinson disease: a model for physical therapy. Physical Therapy, 80:578-597.
103. Murphy R., Tubridy N., Kevelighan H., O'Riordan S.(2013): Parkinson's disease: how is employment affected? Irish Journal of Medical Science, 182(3):415-9.
104. Nieuwboer A., Kwakkel G., Rochester L., Jones D., van Wegen W., Willems A.M., Chavret F., Hetherington V., Baker K., Lim I.(2007): Cueing training in the home improves gait-related mobility in Parkinson's disease: the RESCUE trial. Journal of Neurology, Neurosurgery and Psychiatry, 78:134-140.

105. Nieuwboer A., Weerdt W.D., Dom R., Truyen M., Janssens L., Kamsma Y.(2001): The effect of a home physiotherapy program for persons with Parkinson's disease. Journal of Rehabilitation Medicine, 33(6): 266-72.
106. O'Shea S., Morris M.E., Iansek R.(2002): Dual task interference during gait in people with Parkinson disease: effects of motor versus cognitive secondary tasks. Physical Therapy, 82:888–97.
107. Olanow W.C., Agid Y., Mizuno Y., Albanese U., Damier Ph., de Yebenes J., Gershanik O., Guttman M., Grandas F., Hallet M., Hornykiewicz O., Jenner P., Katzenschlager R., Langston W.J., LeWitt P., Melamed E., Mena M.A., Michel P.P., Mytilineou C., Obeso J.A., Poewe W., Quinn N., Raisman-Vozari R., Rajput A.H., Rascol O., Sampaio C., Stocchi F.(2004): Levodopa in the treatment of Parkinson's disease: current controversies. Movement Disorders, 19(9): 997-1005.
108. Oliveira R.M., Gurd J.M., Nixon P., Marshall J.C., Passingham R.E.(1997): Micrographia in Parkinson's disease: the effect of providing external cues. Journal of Neurology, Neurosurgery and Psychiatry, 63(4):429-433.
109. Pacchetti C., Mancini F., Agheri R., Fundaro C., Martignomi E., Bappi G.(2000): Active music therapy in Parkinson's disease: an integrative method for motor and emotional rehabilitation. Psychosomatic Medicine, 62(3): 386-93.
110. Palmer S., Mortimer J., Webster D., Bistevins B., Dickinson G.(1986): Exercise therapy for Parkinson's disease., Archives of Physical Medicine and Rehabilitation, 67(10):741-745.
111. Paty D., Li W.K.(1993): Interferon beta-1b is effective in relapsing-remitting multiple sclerosis. II. MRI analysis results of a multicenter, randomized, double-blind, placebo-controlled trial. UBC MS/MRI Study Group and the IFNB Multiple Sclerosis Study Group. Neurology, 43(4): 662-667.
112. Paty D.W.(2001): Interferon beta-1b is effective in relapsing-remitting multiple sclerosis. II. MRI analysis results of a multicenter, randomized, double-blind, placebo-controlled trial. 1993 [classical article], Neurology, 57(12 Suppl 5):10-15.
113. Pelissier J., Perennou D.(2000): Reeducation et readaptation des troubles moteurs de la maladie de Parkinson. Revue Neurologique, 156(2):190-200.
114. Pellecchia M.T., Grasso A., Biancardi L.G., Squillante M., Bonavita V., Barone P.(2004): Physical therapy in Parkinson's disease: an open long-term rehabilitation trial. Journal of Neurology, 251 (5):595-598.
115. Platz T., Brown R.G., Marsden C.D.(1998): Training improves the speed of aimed movements in Parkinson's disease. Journal of Neurology, 121(3):505-514.
116. Playfer J.(1999): Parkinson's disease. Postgraduate Medical Journal, 73(859):257-264.
117. Rajput A.H.(2001): Levodopa prolongs life expectancy and is non-toxic to substantia nigra. Parkinsonism and Related Disorders, 8(2):95-100.

118. Ramig L., Countryman S., Thompson L., Horii Y.(1995): Comparison of two forms of intensive treatment for Parkinson's disease. Journal of Speech And Hearing Research, 38(6):1232-1251.
119. Reuter I., Engelhardt M., Stecker K., Baas H.(1999): Therapeutic value of exercise training in Parkinson's disease. Medicine Science Sports Exercise, 31(11):1544-1549.
120. Rochester L., Hetherington V., Jones D., Nieuwboer A., Willems A.M., Kwakkel G., Van Wegen E.(2004): Attending to the task: interference effects of functional tasks on walking in Parkinson's disease and the roles of cognition, depression, fatigue, and balance. Archives of Physical Medicine and Rehabilitation, 85:1578–85.
121. Rochester L, Hetherington V, Jones D, Nieuwboer A., Willems A.M., Kwakkel G., Van Wegen E.(2005): The Effect of External Rhythmic Cues (Auditory and Visual) on Walking During a Functional Task in Homes of People With Parkinson's Disease. Archives of Physical Medicine and Rehabilitation, 86(5):999-1006.
122. Rubinstein T.C., Giladi N., Hausdorff J.M.(2002): The power of cueing to circumvent dopamine deficits: a review of physical therapy treatment of gait disturbances in Parkinson's disease. Movement Disorders, 17:1148-1160.
123. Samii A., Nutt J.G., Ransom B.R.(2004): Parkinson's disease. Lancet, 363:1783-1793.
124. Scandalis T., Bosak A., Berliner J., Helman L., Wells M.(2001): Resistance training and gait function in patients with Parkinson's disease. American Journal of Physical Medicine and Rehabilitation, 80(1):38-43.
125. Schenkman M., Custom M.T., Kuchibhatla M., Chandler J., Pieper C. (1977): Reliability of Impairment and Physical Performance Measure for Persons with Parkinson's disease. Physical Therapy, 77(1):19-27.
126. Schenkman M., Cutson T.M., Kuchibhatla M., Chandler J., Pieper C.F., Ray L., Laub K.C.(1998): Exercise to improve spinal flexibility and function for people with Parkinson's disease: a randomized controlled trial. Journal of The American Geriatrics Society, 46(10):1207-1216.
127. Schenkman M., Donovan J., Tsubota J., Kluss M., Stebbins P., Butler R.B.(1989): Management of individuals with Parkinson's disease: rationale and case studies. Physical Therapy, 69(11):944-55.
128. Schrag A, Banks P.(2006): Time of loss of employment in Parkinson's disease. Movement Disorders, 21(11):1839-43.
129. Schrag A., Jahanshabi M., Quinn N.(2000): What contributes to quality of life in patients with Parkinson's disease? Journal of Neurology, Neurosurgery and Psychiatry, 69(3):308-312.
130. Schultz W., Apilcella P., Romo R., Scamati E.(1995): Context-dependent activity in primate striatum reflecting past and future behavioral events [In:] Houk J.C., Davis J.L., Beiser D.C.(ed.) Models of Information Processing in the Basal Ganglia. Cambridge. Mass: The MIT Press, 11-27.

131. Selby G.(1975): Parkinson's disease. [In:] Vinken P.J., Bruyn G.W.(ed.), Handbook of Clinical Neurology 2nd ed. Amsterdam, the Netherlands: Elsever, 173-211.
132. Shen X., Mak M.(2015): Technology-Assisted Balance and Gait Training Reduces Falls in Patients With Parkinson's Disease: A Randomized Controlled Trial With 12-Month *Follow-up*. Neurorehabilitation and Neural Repair, 29(2):103-111.
133. Shoenberg B.S.(1987): Epidemiology of movement disorders. [In:] Marsden C.D., Fahn S.(ed.): Movement Disorders 2, London, England, Butterworth, 17-32.
134. Sławek J., Lass P., Derejko M., Dubaniewicz M.(2001): Cerebral blood flow SPECT may be helpful in establishing the diagnosis of progressive supranuclear palsy and corticobasal degeneration. Nuclear Medicine Review Central and Eastern Europe, 4:73-76.
135. Snow B.J.(2000): Parkinson's disease and related disorders. [In:] Evans GJ, Williams F, Beattie LB, Michael JP, Wilcock GK [red.]. Oxford Textbook of Geriatric Medicine. Oxford University Press, Oxford.
136. Soliveri P., Brown R., Jaharishahi M., Marsolen C.(1992): Effect of practice on performance of skilled motor task in Parkinson's disease. Journal of Neurology, Neurosurgery, and Psychiatry, 55:454-460.
137. Stack E., Ashburn A.(2005): Early Development of the Standing Start 180 Turn Test. Physiotherapy, 91:6-13.
138. Stallibrass C., Sissons P., Chalmers C.(2002): Randomized controlled trial of the Alexander Technique for idiopathic Parkinson's disease. Clinical Rehabilitation, 16:695-708.
139. Steward C., Winfield L., Hunt A., Bressman S.B., Fahn S., Blitzer A., Brin M.F.(1995): Speech dysfunction in Early Parkinson's disease. Movement Disorders, 10:562-565.
140. Tanner C.M., Langston J.W.(1990): Do environmental toxins cause Parkinson's disease? A critical review. Neurology, 40(suppl.3):17-30.
141. Thacker E.L., Chen H., Patel A.V., McCullough M.L., Calle E.E., Thun M.J., Schwarzschild M.A., Ascherio A.(2008): Recreational physical activity and risk of Parkinson's disease. Movement Disorders, 23(1): 69-74.
142. Thaut M., McIntosh G., Rice R., Miller R., Rathbiun J., Brault J.(1996): Rhythmic auditory stimulation in gait training for Parkinson's disease patients. Movement Disorders, 11(2):193-200.
143. Thomas S., MacMahon D., Henry S.(1999): Moving and Shaping - The Future: Commissioning Services for People with Parkinson's. Parkinson's Society of the United Kingdom, London.
144. Tison F., Barberger-Gateau P., Dubroca B., Henry P., Dartigues J.F.(1997): Dependency in Parkinson's disease: a population-based survey in nondemented elderly subjects. Movement Disorders, 12(6):910-915.
145. Tomlinson C.L., Patel S., Meek C., Herd C.P., Clarke C.E.; Stowe R., Shah L., Sackley C.O., Deane K.H., Wheatley K., Ives N.(2012): Physiotherapy

intervention in Parkinson's disease: systematic review and meta-analysis. BMJ, 345:e5004.
146. Toole R., Hirsch M., Forkink A., Lehman D., Martland C.(2000): The effects of a balance and strength training program on equilibrium in Parkinsonism: a preliminary study. NeuroRehabilitation, 14(3):165-174.
147. Trend P., Kaye J., Gage H., Owen C., Wade D.(2002): Short-term effectiveness of intensive multidisciplinary rehabilitation for people with Parkinson's disease and their carers. Clinical Rehabilitation, 16(7):717-725.
148. Tröster A.I., Paolo A.M., Lyons K.E., Glatt S.L., Hubble J.P., Koller W.C.(1995): The influence of depression on cognition in Parkinson's disease: a pattern of impairment distinguishable from Alzheimer's disease. Neurology, 45(4):672-676.
149. Viliani T., Pasquetti P., Magnolfi S., Lunardelli M.L., Giorgi C., Serra P., Taiti P.G.(1999): Effects of physical training on straightening-up. Disability and Rehabilitation, 21:68-73.
150. Viliani T., Pasquetti P., Magnolfi S., Lunardelli M.L., Giorgi C., Serra P., Taiti P.G.(1999): Effects of physical training on straightening up processes in patients with Parkinson's disease. Disability and Rehabilitation, 21(2):68-73.
151. Wade D., Gage H., Owen C., Trend P., Grossmith G., Kaye J.(2002): Multidisciplinary rehabilitation for people with Parkinson's disease: a randomised controlled study. Journal of Neurology, Neurosurgery and Psychiatry, 74(2):158-162.
152. Wells K.B., Siewerd A., Hays R.D., Burnam A., Rogers W., Daniels M., Berry S.(1989): Results from the Medical Outcome Study. Journal of the American Medical Association, 262:914-919.
153. Wells M.R, Giantinoto S., D'Agate D., Areman R.D., Fazzini E.A., Dowling D., Bosak A.(1999): Standard osteopathic manipulative treatment acutely improves gait performance in patients with Parkinson's disease. Journal of The American Osteopathic Association, 99(2):92-99.
154. WHO, Quality of Life. Special report, (1992).
155. Worringham C., Stelmach G.(1990): Practice effects on the preprogramming of discrete movements in Parkinson's disease. Journal of Neurology, Neurosurgery and Psychiatry, 53(8):702-704.
156. Yogev G., Giladi N., Peretz C., Springer S., Simon E.S., Hausdorff J.M.(2005): Dual tasking, gait rhythmicity, and Parkinson's disease: which aspects of gait are attention demanding? European Journal of Neuroscience, 22:1248–56.
157. Zhang Z.X., Roamn G.C.(1993): Worldwide occurrence of Parkinson's disease: an updated review. Neuroepidemiology, 12:195-208.
158. Zurcher G., Dingemanse J., Da Prada M.(1991): Ro 40–7592, a potent inhibitor of extracerebral and brain catechol-0-methyltransferase: preclinical and clinical findings. [In:] New Developments in Therapy of Parkinson's Disease. Agnoli A., Campanella G.(ed.), John Libbey CIC, Rome, 37-43.

Appendix

Program of the rehabilitation activities

The implementation of activities guided by the following objectives:
1 - in the treatment and rehabilitation of hypokinesia (posture, posture reflexes and reflexes of balance):
The purpose of physical therapy was optimal use of still preserved patterns for acquired and automatic movements. Since one of the elements of PD are impaired ability to learn new patterns of the movement, and it is already present in its early stages, it is impossible to generate new routes and thus learning a new motion system. To achieve favorable results the rehabilitation was guided by the following conditions:
- frequent repetition of movements,
- coupling movements with acoustic initiator of the movement (step),
- repetition of movements with different frequencies,
- the introduction of voluntary movements with the stimulating mechanisms (verbal commands, audio support, tactile stimuli, visual stimuli, imaginative stimulation of the movement before his performance, a combination of head and eye movements together with movements of the limbs and the whole body,
- calling reflexes of balance,
- awareness of incorrect posture and its correction.

2 - the treatment and rehabilitation of stiffness:
Rehabilitation treatment was consisted not so much to combat stiffness, but also to reduce its negative impact. The goal of the procedure was:
- objective assessment of the range of the joints motion,
- visibility in the subjective sense of the improvement of mobility in everyday life,
- reduction of muscle tension,
- reduction of muscle soreness.

3 - rehabilitation proceedings in the case of tremor:
The strategy was to reduce tremor, based on:
- in the case of precise movements such as buttoning buttons, tying shoelaces patient was not under time pressure or not under observation,
- in the case of unilateral tremor, the healthy hand was immobilizing the hand with tremor (dishes with drinks were kept by both hands)
- in the case of writing, forearms were based,
- in the case of feet and legs tremor in a sitting position, the leg was set up behind chair or table leg,
- in the case of unilateral tremor, healthy leg was immobilizing the leg with tremor,
- while standing weight was transferred from one leg to the other, from fingers to the heels, few steps were performed.

Class 1

Warm-up

Rehabilitation treatment of hypokinesia - exercise in a seated position - exercises mobilizing various sections of the spine.

Starting position: sitting on a chair with a backrest.
- Move of the eyes to the right/left and then turn of the head to the right/left, while the patient sticks to firmly seat.
- Slowly turn of the head to the right/left with movements of nods when turning.
- Tilting head left/right, then putting the right/left hand on the head so patient can touch the ear on the opposite side.

Starting position: sitting on a stool, both lower limbs apart.
- With the swing patient grasps with both hands the right/left edge of the seat, as far as possible from the rear. Sight is directed straight ahead.
- Patient shifts weight to the right/left buttock. The raised part of the pelvis is rapidly ejected forward and rearward.
- When turning the torso to the right patient bents the right lower limb and with both hands, he/she claps his/her right thigh. Then the body straightens out and the patient returns to the starting position.
- Rhythmic clapping on the right, front, and left side. Upper limbs are alternately bent and straightened.
- The patient holds the foot based on the seat and as close as possible to the buttocks. Keeps both hands for drumstick. The maximum flexion in the hips and knees should be kept as long as possible to avoid difficulties, for example, during dressing up socks or shoes.
- Bending the right/left lower limb towards the opposite shoulder.

The transition from sitting to standing position

Starting position: sitting on a stool.
- Both feet forward of, the left/right foot is more extended forward. Hands laced placed on the chest. Thanks to the rapid movement of "tipping" of both hands in front and toward to the right/left it becomes possible to raise to a standing position. Through hands gliding back to the chest the seating position on a stool is reached again.
- Right/left foot is extended forward. Both hands are stretched and they hold the edge of the chair on the right/left side. At the command of "swing forward high" patient performs the swing with his/her arms forward, leans forward and raises to a standing position. At the command of "swing back" the shoulders return and sit on a stool position is again.

Walking exercises
- The patient is in the standing position. Patient right/left arm heavily leans forward, on command patient moves the opposite lower limb.
- The patient in the standing position. At the command of "left-right" the patient walks in place. Then, on physiotherapist's command "Now go" the patient starts to go.
- The patient in the standing position. In front of left foot, there is a small obstacle (ball). On command, the patient overcomes an obstacle and starts to move.
- Patient claps right/left hand on the right/left thigh, and thus patient gives a command to perform a step that leg.

The problem of a narrow channel - the entry into the room.

- Corridor formed with (tape, pins, balls, rear backrests of chairs) at various intervals to form the constriction. Patient should pass these corridors without changing the rate or step length.

Independent gait with simultaneous performance of motor programs.
- Rotating the gym ball during gait.
- Throwing up and catching the ball during gait.

Exercise in pairs in a standing position.
- Patients stand sideways to each other holding hands. Abutting the lower limbs perform a forwards and backwards movements. In this exercise, emphasis is placed on the maintenance of bent position.

In the next exercise is required the upright position.
- Participants stand in a circle, arms are straight. They hold hands tightly. Everyone extends right lower limb forward and backward. At the command, change legs.
- On a similar command, hit the floor with the right/left foot at the front, right and left rear of the feet of the loaded lower limb. Change loaded legs.

Calming Exercises

Class 2

Warm-up
Exercises in straight sitting position - rehabilitation treatment of hypokinesia.
- The patient sits in inclined rearwards position based on the upper limbs that are set in abducted position with external rotation. Lower limbs are lightly abducted. Lift right/left hip.
- The patient in the same position of the arms, carries the momentum of right/left lower limb on the opposite side, until patient lift the hip.
- The patient sits leaning with both hands on the right/left side. Patient tries to abduct the lower limb on the opposite side.
- Lower limb on the opposite side is briefly raised.
- Upper limbs are facing forward, hands are clenched. Both lower limbs are slightly apart. The patient takes a strong turn of the shoulder girdle and upper limb to the right/left, looking for the path of movement.
- In a similar position and with identical upper limb movement towards the right/left, left/right lower limb moves forward.

Exercises designed to: improve posture, calling the reflexes of balance, posture awareness abnormal posture and its correction.
Exercises in a standing position with support.
- The patient is standing sideways to the ladder gym. Both hands hold a rung high above patient's head. The feet are close to the last rung. It stretches the back side muscles, by bending the torso to the right/left.
- The patient being in a similar position, carries a maximum twist of the torso so that patient touches the ladder gym once with back and once with belly.
- The patient stands with his face to the ladder gym, holding rung with upper limbs with straight elbows, as high as possible. Then, patient tries to swing the torso as far as possible from ladders gym.
- A patient in a similar starting position tilt torso to rear and make moves of his/her hips to the right and left.
- In a similar starting position, the patient sets the lower limbs wide apart and practices weight shifting from left foot to the right.
- Accelerating and enhancing the lateral transfer of body weight by lifting up the unloaded lower limb.
- Facing the ladder gym, the patient holds rung at shoulder level with both hands. Then, on the command patient begins to tread in place.
- On the command "stop" patient stops treading and stays in such a way that one lower limb is loaded and the other is unloaded.
- On the command "to the right" or "to the left", the feet are moved so that the lower part of the torso is twisted to the right/left, while its upper part due to sticking patient's hands at rung at the shoulder level remains in frontal position.

Exercises to overcome the resistance to the initiation of movement while solidify - "freezing".
The weight of the body rests on the entire surface of the foot.
- Move the weight from one leg to the other (swinging). Then do step forward with unloaded leg.
- Try to make the first step to the side, or backward.
- Pat the thigh.

- Pull the arm straight ahead and try to reach to it knee.
- Give yourself loud command, for example, one - two, knee up, etc.
- Use the marks found on the floor.

Calming exercises

Class 3

Warm-up
Exercise to reduce stiffness.
Starting position: sitting on a stool.
- Light spacing of the legs, the pelvis is set in slight flexion, relaxed hands resting on the shoulders. Rotating body to the right and to the left.
- The same exercise only with an intense twist the torso.
- Right/left upper limb rests freely on the left/right knee. The coup of the left/right shoulder in the front and back.
- A similar exercise, the patient looks at the movement of arms.
- Arm swings forward and backward. Emphasis is placed on the swing arm in front up to shoulder level.
- A similar exercise. The emphasis is on swing both arms backwards.
- Turn the torso to the right/left. Patient moves and swing both upper limbs backward and forward on one side - the right/left.
- The torso is upright. Both hands make swinging moves back and forth. During the forward movement of the arms pivot outwards, and during the backward swing of the arms the pivot inward (thumbs pointing inwards).
- The arms are at shoulder level. Right arm to the front, left to the back. The movements of both arms swinging up to head level. The upper part of the body also performs twist move.
- Both arms are resting on the head, elbows are directed sideways. Patient turns the torso to the right/left. The head remains in the straight ahead position (it should not be accompanied by movement of pelvis and legs).
- The patient performs arm swings sideways, over his head up to clap.
- Both arms perform swing motion in the sagittal plane. Patient claps his hands in the front and in the back.
- Both legs are wide apart. During exhalation body is leaning forward and resting on one of the lower limbs, upper limbs performe swinging back and forth.
- Sitting on a chair patient crossed his legs and performs feet spinning left/right and change legs.
Exercises with ladders gym for hypokinesia.
- The patient stands facing the ladder gym. He keeps his upper limbs with elbows straight on the rung below the level of the shoulders. Body weight is transferred to the right/left lower limb. During this time the unloaded leg perform swinging moves parallel to the ladder gym, forward and backward.
- Standing right/left side of the ladder gym in stride position. With his right hand patient is holding the ring at the shoulder girdle level. Body weight transfers to the front extended lower limb and returns back to the starting position.
- Moving forward center of gravity can be even more intensified by rising a little of the unloaded lower limb.
- In a similar starting position, the patient moves his weight backwards and consciously return to the starting position.
- In a similar starting position, a rapid change of the center of gravity forward and backward. Then conscious return to the starting point on both feet evenly loaded.
Calming exercises

Class 4

Warm-up
Stretching, strengthening exercises- a position of lying back.
- Both upper limbs are under the head, right/left lower limb is straight, left/right lower limb is bent at the knee. The pelvis on the bent side of the lower limb is lifted up to the extension in the hip.
- Both lower limbs are bent, lift the pelvis up and slight movement from side to side.
- The change in the right/left lower limb bending and extension shoving on the floor; gradually increasing the pace.
-Bent of both lower limbs. The lateral surfaces of the feet touch the floor, adduction and abduction of the knee.
- The right/left lower limb slump up outside and bring back.
- Both hands are resting flat on the ribs curves and move together with the chest during breathing; inhale/exhale through the mouth through the nose. During exhalation patient should pronounce consonant 'p', 't', 'k', 'f'.

Exercises in lying ahead position.
- Both upper limbs are arranged under the forehead. Patient lifts right/left lower limb up while lifting the right/left hip.
- Both upper limbs are straight arranged over head. Right/left lower limb is bent sideways at the hip and knee. At the same time the patient turns his head toward the bent lower limb. Then patient straightens lower limb and turns back his head.

Exercises in standing position - walking.
- The patient walks in the place and at every step he lifts the knee up. Hands perform free movements.
- Walking in the place the patient takes a few steps to the side and back, at the end of this exercise spins in a circle.
- Walking on the track corresponding to the shape of the letter.
- Walking along the rays of the stars arranged with tape.
- Two ropes were laid on the floor (tape), in the initial section of the narrow and diverging. At the end there is the ball. It is important to raise the leg when crossing over the ball.
- On the floor lies a cardboard box. The patient sets behind it. Raises one foot over it. On the other side carefully puts foot on the floor in front of cardboard starting from the heel to the toes. Then it moves back behind the cardboard. Change legs.
- The patient is on the side of the cardboard box and several times he/she passes to the other side.
Calming exercises.

The program of the rehabilitation for the patient at home

Remember!
Morning gymnastics has irreplaceable value. If you want to succeed in physical therapy, then regularity of exercise is necessary. Therefore, regardless of the therapy - alone at home perform daily exercises.

Remember of the correct posture.

Stand back next to the wall or the door, straighten up and try to push to the surface of the walls your head (occiput), shoulders, arms and hips. Ask your family to draw the attention to maintaining good posture.

Walking exercises.

Walk in the place and with each step lift the knee up. Remember of balancing one and the other hand, look ahead (not at feet). Do a few steps to the side (both sides). When doing this exercise primarily watch to keep your back straight and keep balance.

Stretching exercises.

Stand at a table with your hands resting on the table (fingers straight). Try to straighten the arm at the elbows joints and then move your weight forward - it increases the muscle stretch.

Stand against a wall. Hands adhere to the walls, the fingers and elbows are straight and direct fingertips toward the ceiling. Very slowly move your hands on the wall toward to the floor. Try to hold this position for 10 seconds. Then move your hands toward the ceiling. Try to hold this position for 10 seconds.
Remember - the feeling of stretching should not be painful!

Exercise arms.

Standing - lift the arms to the level and clap over your head then lower the arms to behind the back and clap on the back of the torso.

Exercise feet.

Sit on a stool. Leaving the toes on the floor, lift and lower the heels, hitting them on the floor. Then, leaving the heel on the floor, lift and lower the toes and hitting by forefoot on the floor.

Exercise of manual dexterity.

Sit on a stool. Put your hands on your thighs, and then fairly quickly pick them up and knock on the thigh for a change - a volar and dorsal surface, turning the palms.
Open hands - straighten your fingers, close your hands – clench your fingers.

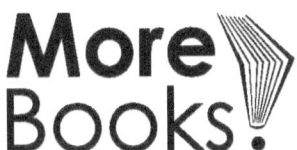
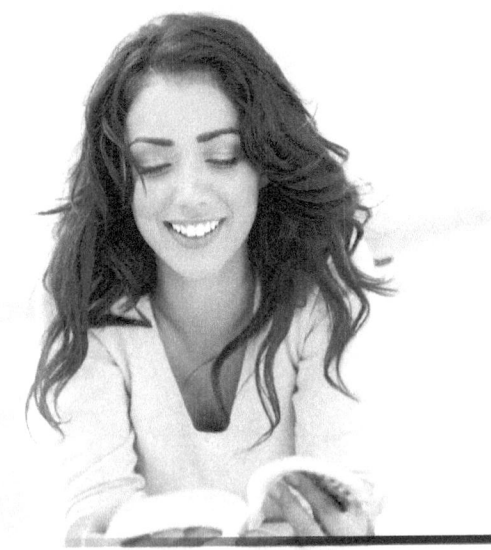

I want morebooks!

Buy your books fast and straightforward online - at one of the world's fastest growing online book stores! Environmentally sound due to Print-on-Demand technologies.

Buy your books online at
www.get-morebooks.com

Kaufen Sie Ihre Bücher schnell und unkompliziert online – auf einer der am schnellsten wachsenden Buchhandelsplattformen weltweit!
Dank Print-On-Demand umwelt- und ressourcenschonend produziert.

Bücher schneller online kaufen
www.morebooks.de

OmniScriptum Marketing DEU GmbH
Heinrich-Böcking-Str. 6-8
D - 66121 Saarbrücken
Telefax: +49 681 93 81 567-9

info@omniscriptum.com
www.omniscriptum.com

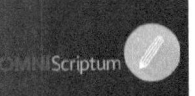

www.ingramcontent.com/pod-product-compliance
Lightning Source LLC
Chambersburg PA
CBHW031536210526
45464CB00003B/1030